Beyond Benzos
Benzo Addiction, Benzo Withdrawal, and Long-term Recovery from Benzodiazepines

by Taite Adams

Rapid Response Press
1730 Lighthouse Terr. S., Suite 12
So Pasadena, FL 33707
www.rapidresponsepress.com
Ordering Information:
Quantity sales. Special discounts are available on quantity purchases by corporations, associations, and others. For details, contact the publisher at the address above.
Orders by U.S. trade bookstores and wholesalers. Please contact Rapid Response Press: Tel: (866) 983-3025; Fax: (855) 877-4736 or visit www.rapidresponsepress.com.
Printed in the United States of America
Publisher's Cataloging-in-Publication data
Adams, Taite.
A title of a book : a subtitle of the same book / Taite Adams.
p. cm.
ISBN 978-0-9907674-3-5
1. The main category of the book —Health —Other category. 2. Another subject category —Mind and Body. 3. More categories —Recovery.

First Edition
==================

Limit of Liability/Disclaimer of Warranty

Limit of Liability/Disclaimer of Warranty: While the publisher and author have used their best efforts in preparing this book, they make no representations or warranties with respect to the accuracy or completeness of the contents of this book and specifically disclaim any implied warranties or merchantability or fitness for a particular purpose. No warranty may be created or extended by sales representatives or written sales materials. The advice and strategies contained herein may not be suitable for your situation. You should consult with a professional where appropriate. The publisher and author do not assume and hereby disclaim any liability to any party for any loss, damage, or disruption caused by errors or omissions, whether such errors or omissions result from negligence, accident, or any other cause.

================

Disclaimer

Disclaimer: This publication is designed to provide accurate and personal experience information in regard to the subject matter covered. It is sold with the understanding that the author, contributors, publisher are not engaged in rendering counseling or other professional services. If counseling advice or other expert assistance is required, the services of a competent professional person should be sought out.

==================

Medical Disclaimer

The information contained in this book is not intended to serve as a replacement for professional medical advice. Any use of the information in this book is at the reader's discretion. The author and publisher specifically disclaim any and all liability arising directly or indirectly from the use or application of any information contained in this book. A health care professional should be consulted regarding your specific situation.

To Mom - This one is for you. You can do this;

To my son - Stay away from xans, bars, and kpins. I love you;

To my love - Life with you is as it should be - pure joy.

See http://www.TaiteAdams.com
for more info

Table of Contents

Preface

All great changes are preceded by chaos. – Deepak Chopra

Termed by some as the world's deadliest pill, the class of prescription drugs known as Benzodiazepines are on the cusp of racing past opiates to earn the label as this nation's most widely abused class of drugs. As it is, Xanax remains the world's most popular pill, with prescriptions for it and other benzos going up 12% per year. While long thought to be harmless medication for a wide variety of ailments, this is the furthest thing from the truth. With my own personal experience with Benzodiazepine addiction on several fronts, I know this to be the case.

In just ten years, the instances of benzo-related hospital admissions has increased over 500%, with half of those being admitted reporting daily benzodiazepine use. While many who use these medications, illicitly or otherwise, do so in combination with other drugs, the fact remains that benzos are highly addictive and incredibly difficult to get off of. I, personally, took benzos in combination with opiate painkillers for years. I was addicted to both and didn't know enough about either drug to be terrified of detox when the time came. I should have been. I have a parent who unwittingly became addicted to Ativan after years of use and continues to fight that difficult battle back into the light.

Are there legitimate uses for benzos? There are but that isn't what this book is about and, if you are trying to justify your continuing use of these dangerous medications, you should probably search out another book for that purpose. I can't help you with that. However, if benzos have taken over your life or that of someone close to you, this is something that I am intimately familiar with and we have a lot to discuss.

What are Benzos?

The largest part of what we call 'personality' is determined by how we've opted to defend ourselves against anxiety and sadness.
— Alain de Botton

Benzodiazepines are a class of psychoactive drugs that produce central nervous system (CNS) depression and that are most commonly used to treat anxiety and insomnia. Benzodiazepines are some of the most common medications in the world; a recent study sponsored by the National Institutes of Health found that about 1 in 20 adults received a prescription for them in 2008. Over 150 million prescriptions for these drugs are written annually in this country alone.

Story:

With no history of addiction, Jane went to a psychiatrist in 1994 due to pressures at work. He immediately put her on 0.5 mg/day Klonopin and then increased her dose to 3mg/day, even though she didn't ask for more. When she finally hit severe tolerance withdrawal 3 years later, he indicated that he thought she might be "partying with friends", even though she was in her 50's. Jane tried to quit cold turkey and ended up in the ER. Since, she has landed in detox, support group meetings, has lost her job, her family, and her dignity. All of this from a legal prescription from a trusted physician

Benzodiazepine History

The natural role of twentieth-century man is anxiety. - Norman Mailer

In the early to mid 1900's, America began a love affair with various synthetic barbiturates out of Germany that were marketed under different names such as Secanol and Luminal, and were touted as the cures for anxiety and insomnia. By the time the U.S. entered World War II, we were consuming nearly a billion of these little pills annually and addiction had become an epidemic. This is where the term "goofballs" came from with regards to the deadly combo of barbiturates and alcohol. These drugs became very dangerous with some high profile OD's, notably Marilyn Monroe and Judy Garland. In 1951, legislation was passed making these sorts of drugs prescription only and giving the impression that the danger was over and physician supervision was the answer. It definitely was not.

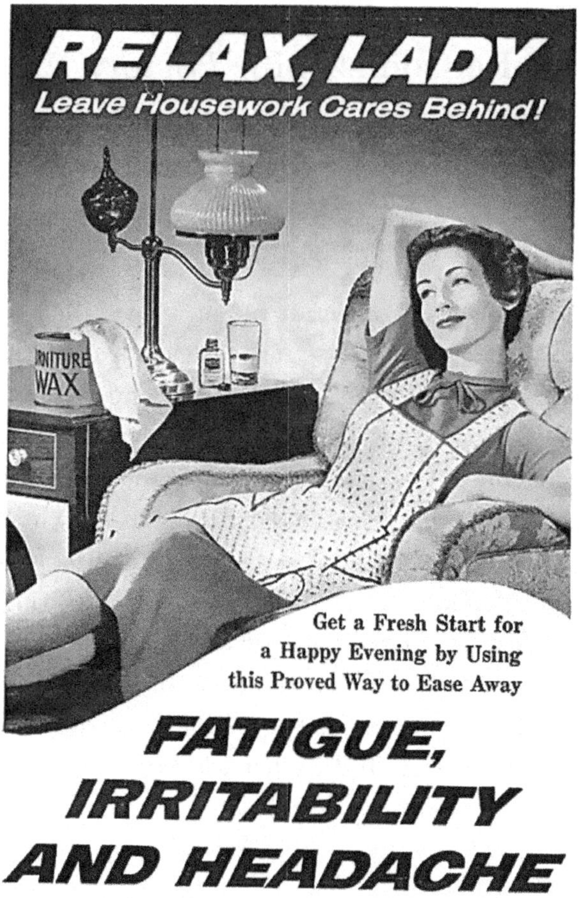

As barbiturates faded into the background, the first benzodiazepine (Librium) was patented in 1960 by Hoffmann-LaRoche. Not long after, the same company began marketing Valium and, by 1977, benzos were the most globally prescribed medication. As early as 1979, Sen. Ted Kennedy called a Senate Health subcommittee hearing on the dangers of benzodiazepines in which he said the drugs "produced a nightmare of dependence and addiction, both very difficult to treat and recover from." Yet, sadly, little was acknowledged or done. While over 2,000 different benzodiazepines have been produced, only about 15 are currently FDA-approved in the United States and they are classified according to how long their effects last.

Different Kinds of Benzos

Again, there are many different kinds of benzos and they are classified, in most countries, according to their potency and the speed with which they metabolize, or their half-life. Here is a list of the most common benzodiazepines, along with their trade names.

- **Alprazolam (Xanax)** - FDA approved for the treatment of panic and anxiety disorders. Alprazolam is the most prescribed benzodiazepine in the U.S.

- **Bromazepam (Lectopam)** - Used as a short-term treatment for anxiety and to alleviate anxiety before surgery.

- **Brotizolam (Lendormin)** - A very potent anxiolytic, hypnotic, and anticonvulsant drug with fast onset of action. It is used to treat severe insomnia. The drug is not approved in Canada, Britain and the U.S.

- **Chlordiazepoxide (Librium)** - Used for the management of alcohol withdrawal syndrome.

- **Clonazepam (Klonopin)** - A high potency sedative, anxiolytic, hypnotic, and anti-convulsant drug. Clonazepam is a long acting benzodiazepine with a half life between 20 to 50 hours. The FDA has approved the drug for treatment of epilepsy and panic disorder.

- **Clorazepate (Tranxene)** - A hypnotic, sedative, anxiolytic drug used to treat severe insomnia and anxiety disorders.

- **Clotiazepam (Clozan)** - Used for short term anxiety treatment.

- **Cloxazolam (Sepazon)** - Prescribed to treat anxiety.
- **Diazepam (Valium)** - An anxiolytic, hypnotic, sedative, and anticonvulsant drug with rapid onset. It is used to treat panic attacks, insomnia, seizures, restless leg syndrome, and alcohol withdrawal. Diazepam is also used for the treatment of benzodiazepine dependence because of its low potency.
- **Estazolam (ProSom)** - A sedative, anxiolytic drug prescribed for short term treatment of insomnia
- **Etizolam (Etilaam)** - Used to treat insomnia
- **Flunitrazepam (Rohypnol)** - Usually prescribed for short term treatment of chronically severe insomnia. The drug is sometimes misused as a date rape drug because of its ability to cause amnesia.
- **Flurazepam (Dalmane)** - A sedative, anxiolytic drug used to treat mild to moderate insomnia.
- **Loprazolam (Somnovit)** - A sedative, anxiolytic drug used to treat moderately severe insomnia.
- **Lorazepam (Ativan)** - A very high-potent drug with sedative, anxiolytic, and muscle relaxation properties. It is prescribed for the short-term management of severe anxiety.
- **Midazolam (Dormicum)** - A high potent drug with anxiolytic, amnestic, hypnotic, anticonvulsant, skeletal muscle relaxant, and sedative properties. It is used to treat acute seizures and severe insomnia, as well as inducing sedation before surgical procedures.
- **Nitrazepam (Alodorm)** - A hypnotic drug used to treat severe insomnia.

- **Nordazepam (Nordaz)** - An anticonvulsant, anxiolytic, muscle relaxant and sedative drug used to treat anxiety.
- **Oxazepam (Seresta)** - Used to treat anxiety and insomnia and control the symptoms of alcohol withdrawal.
- **Temazepam (Restoril)** - Approved for the short-term treatment of insomnia.
- **Triazolam (Apo-Triazo, Halcion, Hypam, and Trilam)** - Only used as a sedative to treat severe insomnia

Still unsure about their classifications and actions? Here is some more data the breaks down the most widely prescribed drugs:

- **Ultra-short acting** - Midazolam (Versed), Triazolam (Halcion)
- **Short-acting** - Alprazolam (Xanax), Lorazepam (Ativan)
- **Long-acting** - Chlordiazepoxide (Librium), Diazepam (Valium)

We will be discussing half-lifes and their meanings again later on, so if you don't understand the differences in these medications yet, that's ok. Suffice it to say that these distinctions are used in many places for regulatory purposes. For example, a majority of benzos are classified as Schedule IV controlled substances in the United States. The only exception is Rohypnol, which is also Schedule IV but has Schedule I penalties for abuse. Internationally, benzos are also Schedule IV in most places but do have variations in some countries, with the UK putting a few into Schedule III status.

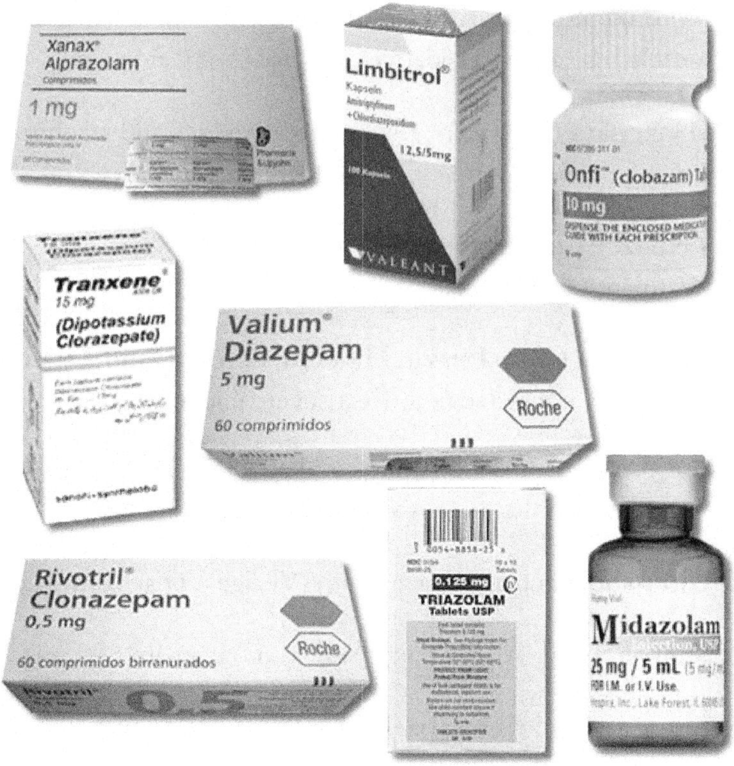
Xanax®
Alprazolam
1 mg
Limbitrol®
Kapseln
12,5/5mg
VALEANT
Onfi™ (clobazam)
10 mg
Tranxene
15 mg
(Dipotassium
Clorazepate)
Valium®
Diazepam
5 mg
60 comprimidos
Roche
Rivotril®
Clonazepam
0,5 mg
60 comprimidos birranurados
Roche
0.125 mg
TRIAZOLAM
Tablets USP
Midazolam
25 mg / 5 mL
FOR I.M. or I.V. Use

How Benzos Work

Medical research has made such progress, that there are practically no healthy people any more. - Aldous Huxley

---

Benzodiazepines work by affecting the way certain brain chemicals transmit messages to certain brain cells. Now that we've been vague, let's get more specific. Benzos work by binding to a receptor which is located on neurons in the brain called the GABA receptor. GABA is a neurotransmitter in the brain and it controls excitability of neurons. Depending upon the action of the particular benzo, as they differ slightly, there are a variety of effects that are produced by the binding to the GABA receptor. These effects include:

- Impaired motor coordination
- Drowsiness, lethargy, fatigue
- Impaired thinking and memory
- Confusion
- Depression
- Altered vision
- Slurred speech, stuttering
- Vertigo
- Tremors
- Respiratory depression

- Nausea, constipation, dry mouth, abdominal discomfort, loss of appetite, vomiting, diarrhea
- Slowed reflexes
- Mood swings
- Hostile and erratic behavior
- Euphoria

This is a pretty wide range of effects and it's clear that results vary depending upon which type of benzo you are prescribed and your dosage. For example, impaired memory is much more common with a very short acting benzo such as Rohypnol (the date rape drug), yet can happen with others.

Benzodiazepines are prescribed to treat a wide range of issues, such as:

- **Generalized anxiety disorder (GAD)** - Benzodiazepines are often used in the treatment of GAD. The National Institute of Health and Clinical Excellence (NICE) recommends the use of benzodiazepines for short term GAD treatment for no longer than one month. SSRIs are considered to be more effective at treating long-term GAD.
- **Insomnia** - As Benzodiazepines can lead to dependence, they are normally only used as a short-term treatment for severe insomnia or on an "irregular/as-needed" basis.
- **Seizures** - Benzodiazepines are powerful anticonvulsants and are very effective at preventing prolonged convulsive epileptic seizures. In fact, when benzos were first introduced, they were strongly promoted as treatment for all forms of epilepsy. This isn't the case any longer but they are still used for various forms

of seizure treatment. The first-line hospital choices for treating seizures are either clonazepam, diazepam, or lorazepam.

- **Alcohol withdrawal** - The most common benzodiazepine prescribed for alcohol withdrawal is chlodiazepoxide, followed by diazepam. The drugs help alcoholics with detoxification and reduce their risk of severe alcohol withdrawal effects. A study conducted at the University of Ioannina School of Medicine in Greece found that people given benzodiazepines were 84 percent less likely to have alcohol withdrawal-related seizures compared to those given placebos. There is quite a danger here, though, of giving people who are addicted to alcohol another addictive substance to cope with withdrawal symptoms. More on that later.

- **Panic attacks** - Because of their rapid anti-anxiety effects, benzodiazepines are very effective at treating anxiety associated with panic disorder. The American Psychiatric Association says that their use for initial treatment is strongly supported by many different study trials. However, UK based NICE says that long-term use of benzodiazepines for the treatment of panic disorder is not recommended.

- **Muscle relaxant** - Benzodiazepines have strong muscle relaxing properties and have been used with some neurologic disturbances, for relief of muscle spasms, and prior to various surgical procedures.

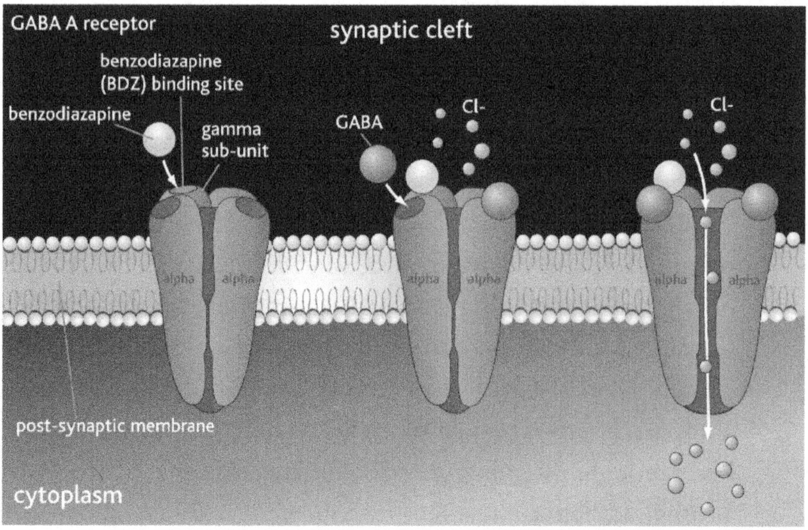

Benzos are administered in a variety of ways but, for the most part, they are manufactured and consumed in pill form. However, they are also available as suppositories and IV injection. When taken orally, they are absorbed through the gastrointestinal tract and then they pass through the liver before exerting action on the rest of the body. Those who use benzos illicitly may ingest them in a variety of ways, such as crushing and snorting pills, injecting pills, smoking and sublingual administration. All of these are dangerous beyond belief and effects vary based upon the type of benzo ingested and the dosage.

The toxicology of these drugs gives an idea of both how quickly the onset of the effects occur and how long the drug takes to metabolize out of your system, or the drug's half-life. Drugs with a short-half life, such as Lorazepam, will require more frequent re-dosing and will produce withdrawal symptoms quicker once use is discontinued. While half-life knowledge might arm you with information to help you pass that next employment drug test, that's not really what this book is aiming to do. The idea here is to impart to you as much information about these drugs as possible. Besides, if you've been taking benzos for a prolonged period of time, chances are that you are hooked and that ship has sailed anyway. Here is some data on the various onset times and drug half-lifes (in hours) of the most common benzos:

Table 1. Common Benzodiazepines, Their Half-lives, and Speeds of Onset

Drug (Brand)	Half-life, h	Speed of Onset
Alprazolam (Niravam, Xanax, Xanax XR, generic)	12-15	Intermediate
Lorazepam (Ativan, Lorazepam Intensol, generic)	10-20	Intermediate
Diazepam (Diastat, Diazepam Intensol, Valium generic)	20-80	Fast
Nordiazepam[a]	31-97	N/A
Oxazepam (Generic)	5-10	Slow
Temazepam (Restoril, generic)	3-13	Fast
Clonazepam (Klonopin, generic)	18-50	Slow

[a]Nordiazepam is not a prescribed drug in the US. It is, however, a metabolite of the following drugs: chlordiazepoxide (Librium), clorazepate (Tranxene), diazepam, halazepam (not available in the US), medazepam, prazepam and tetraprazepam. Based on reference 6.

Story:

Lori was prescribed Ativan (Lorazepam) for just 5 weeks to help with severe insomnia after a kidney stone that required two surgeries. The kidney stone and ureter blockages that she suffered were nothing compared to the pain and discomfort that ensued from Ativan withdrawal. Even 14 months free of the drug, she still suffers withdrawal symptoms and was not on benzos for a prolonged period of time like many.

Benzos and Big Pharma

If there's a pill, then pharmaceutical companies will find a disease for it. - Jeremy Laurance, The Independent

When there is an addiction epidemic of the sort that we are now recognizing with benzodiazepines, the first inclination is to look for someone to blame. I know that when I wrote about "Opiate Addiction", pointing the finger at big pharma wasn't difficult. It's not rocket science here either. The fact of the matter is that, when the myriad of psychotropic drugs came on the market over 50 years ago that appeared to cure everything from schizophrenia to depression to anxiety, the physicians wanted to believe in them as much as the patients and their families. What we can't seem to bring to the light, even today, is that the real truth has been known about these drugs for decades and yet they continue to be prescribed with abandon.

Is this really an industry woven through with corruption? Sadly, it's worse than one could imagine. In years past, new drugs were discovered and brought to market by scientists, chemists, and pharmacologists. Now, they are brought to market by MBA's and marketing gurus. In fact, if there isn't a disorder, or market, for a particular new drug, they will do their best to create one. This very thing was done with Xanax. Its maker, UpJohn, actually coined the phrase "Panic Disorder" and a group of psychiatrists, many with financial ties to the company, went through the process of updating the Diagnostic and Statistical Manual (DSM III) to include this new official diagnosis. According to the Anxiety and Depression Association of America's (ADAA) numbers, there are currently over 6 million people in this country with that diagnosis.

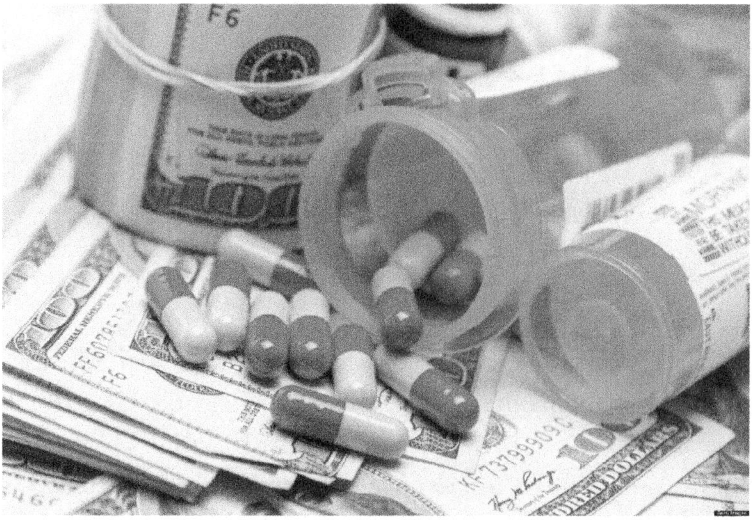

It is widely understood in the medical profession that, when there is a cross-tolerance between substances, the mode of action of those substances is similar. For example, it was known that barbiturates and alcohol had similar action and it had become clear that both were pretty darn addictive. However, when the similarities between the newly-developed benzodiazepines and barbiturates started to surface, both physicians and the pharmaceutical companies by and large made the choice to ignore this and replace one evil with another. (Other substances that bind to the GABA receptor include barbiturates and alcohol.) Benzos were instead touted as the "wave of the future".

Big Pharma has evolved to influence, not only the prescribing physician, but the ultimate consumers as well. While physicians are wined, dined and "hosted" at exotic locales for conferences, they are not supposed to be influenced in any way by these perks. If that rang true, those drug companies would not go to the expense of such extravagance. Additionally, carefully designed drug trials are sponsored by hand-picked physicians and most are anything but scientific or un-biased in their reporting. In 2008, the New York Times reported that a survey of the six top medical journals showed than on average almost 8% of the bylined articles were ghostwritten by freelance writers, then published under the names of cooperating doctors and researchers to give the pro-drug messages contained in the articles the appearance of impartiality.

A 2014 joint investigation by The Milwaukee Journal Sentinel and MedPage Today reviewed a host of ads that often made questionable claims about tranquilizers, stating that they were good for ailments including menopause, gastrointestinal problems, ulcers, and cardiovascular symptoms. In the case of benzodiazepines, institutionalized dispensing of the drugs over the years continues to be linked to promotional activities of drug companies. A 1985 Xanax ad in *JAMA* claimed the drug relieved cardiovascular symptoms -- a claim for which there was no evidence.

Even today there is no rigorous research indicating that Xanax or other benzodiazepines reduce the risk of heart attacks, strokes, or heart disease, said James Stein, MD, professor of medicine and director of preventive cardiology at the University of Wisconsin School of Medicine and Public Health. Stein noted that doctors who were in medical school in 1985 may have seen those ads and formed lasting beliefs that benzodiazepines are beneficial for the heart. "If you learned early in your career, even subliminally, that these drugs were good for the heart or blood vessels, there's an inclination to reach for them," he said. Pfizer, which sells Xanax, declined to provide a comment on the ad.

In the 1970s, ads for the benzodiazepine Librium claimed it was beneficial for ulcers. One such ad in the *New England Journal of Medicine* said the drug was suitable for extended therapy. However, a search of the medical literature turned up no rigorous research showing that Librium cured or reduced the severity of ulcers. "There is no study that shows ulcer healing with anti-anxiolytics (tranquilizers)," said Mitch Roslin, MD, a bariatric surgeon at Lenox Hill Hospital in New York. He said benzodiazepines were used for ulcers based on the theory that anxious people with type A personalities could benefit by reducing their anxiety. A spokesperson for Roche USA, the manufacturer of the drug, said the company couldn't provide a source to give historical perspective on the marketing of its drugs during that time.

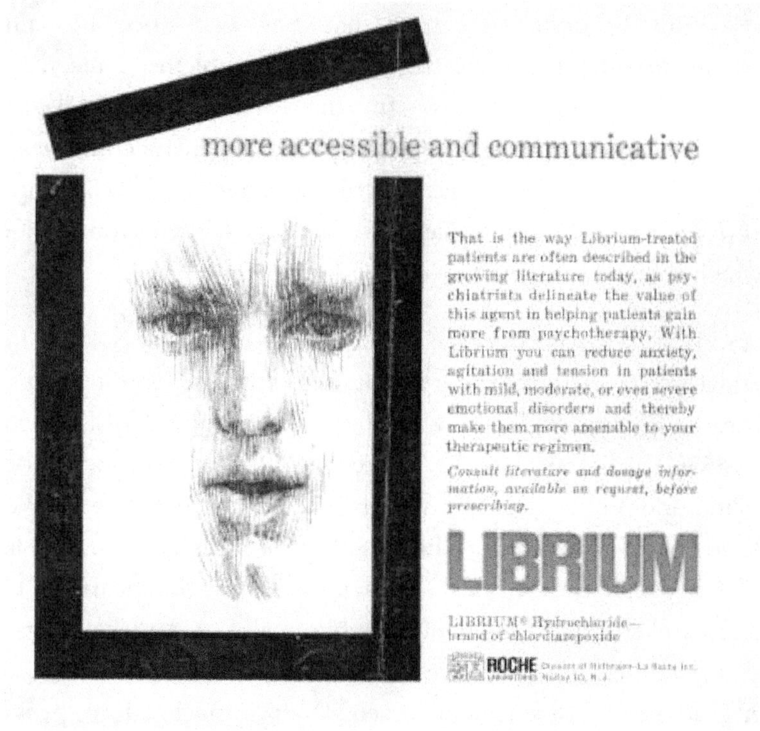

An industry so important to public health and so heavily subsidized and protected by government has social responsibilities that should not be totally overshadowed by its drive for profits. - Dr M. Angell New England Journal of Medicine

The UK seems to be a step ahead with regards to fighting back, having been the host to the largest-ever class-action lawsuit against drug manufacturers in the 1980's and early 1990's, involving 14,000 patients that alleged the manufacturers knew of the dependency potential of the drug but intentionally withheld the information from doctors. At the same time, 117 physicians and 50 health authorities were also sued to recover the harmful effects of dependence and withdrawal.

Are the patients completely free of blame? Like it or not, consumers have been hit with direct advertisements from drug companies for years that have convinced them that certain medications are the cure-all for whatever ails them. This can put a physician in a tough corner when a patient storms their office, armed with 100+ pages of WebMD printouts and drug trial reports, demanding that they be given a prescription for a certain medication. Not to mention, those patients who skip the physician appointment altogether and simply jump online to an internet pharmacy to get their wishes granted.

Now that we can see the various paths to our present state, what does it really matter? It doesn't because benzo addiction places everyone in the same place, no matter what path they took to get there.

Benzo Addiction

Going to a psychiatrist has become one of the most dangerous things a person can do. - Peter Breggin, MD

I've written quite a few books about addiction in past several years. While I have been quick to acknowledge my alcoholism and incredibly serious opiate addiction, one thing that I haven't discussed was my addiction to benzos. While I obtained my opiate painkillers in an after-market, and felonious, manner, I justified my continued daily Xanax use because those meds were prescribed by a legitimate physician. The fact is that it made no difference. I was taking the drugs on a daily basis, just like the other ones, and I was hopelessly hooked.

I don't know about you, but I always had this image in my mind of the quintessential drug addict and it wasn't the one that I saw in the mirror each morning. However, if you're feeling the same way, it always makes me feel better to know that this disease (and it IS a disease) doesn't discriminate and that being addicted to benzos actually puts me in some pretty exclusive company.

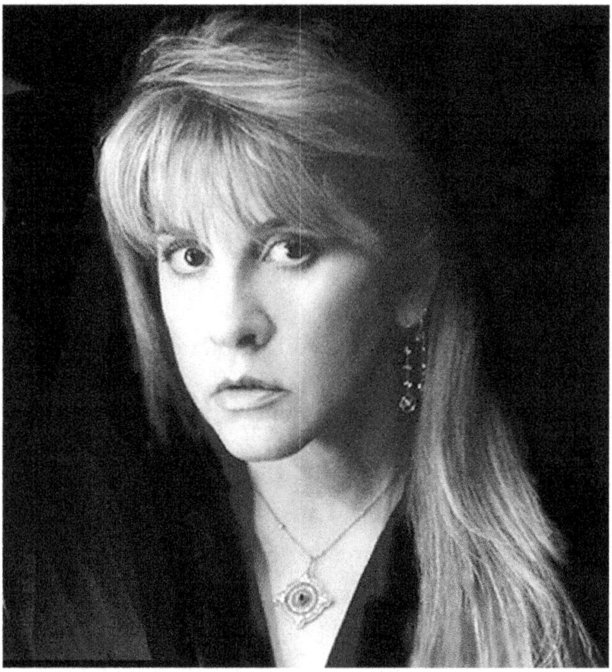

In 1986, Seventies rock star Stevie Nicks checked herself into the Betty Ford Clinic for treatment of cocaine addiction. It was after leaving there that she was first prescribed benzos by a psychiatrist to "help with her sobriety". What followed was 8 years of hell and a horrific detox. "Klonopin is a horrible, dangerous drug," says Nicks, an addict for eight years. "Doctors are dying to put you on drugs: 'Feeling a little nervous? Here, let's mask everything so you don't have a personality anymore.'" Of the celebrities that have overdosed on drugs in recent years, the number with benzodiazepines in their systems are staggering. Among them are: Philip Seymour Hoffman, Whitney Houston, Heath Ledger, Amy Winehouse, Brittany Murphy, and Michael Jackson.

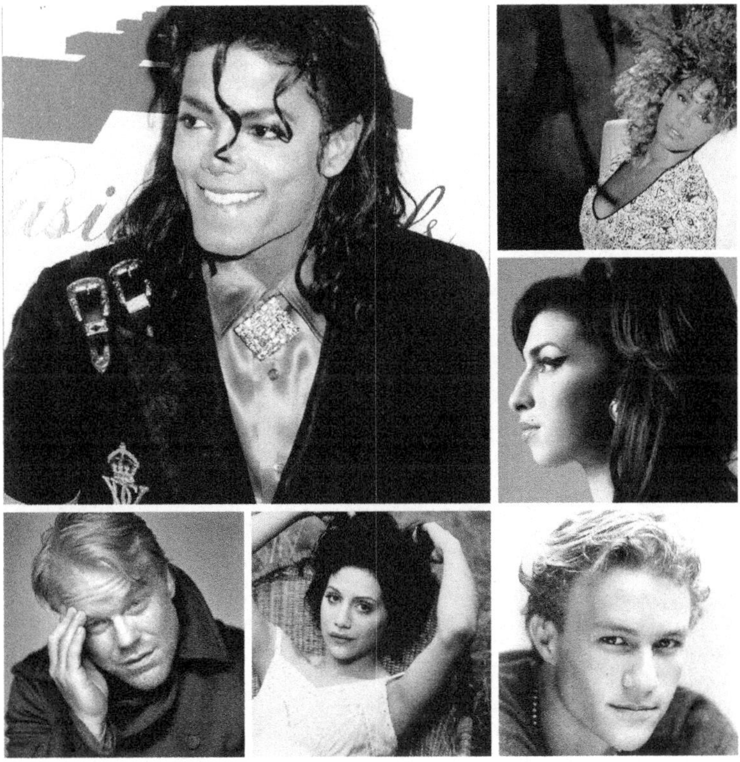

The Addiction vs. Dependency Argument

Increasing numbers of people have been turned into drug addicts through legal prescriptions which perhaps suits the politicians and multi-national bureaucrats as well as the drug companies for it ensures an uncomplaining and docile community which is easy to administer, manage and manipulate...tranquillizers are more addictive than heroin. - Dr Vernon Coleman

---

The term "accidental addict" has become popular in recent years to refer to those people who became addicted to various prescription drugs that were initially prescribed to them by a trusted physician. Depending on who is making use of the term at any given time, the circumstances then vary widely between the housewife who continues to take the pills as prescribed and then finds that she can't get off of them to the person who later resorts to doctor-shopping and buying the drugs on the street to "get by". This is a BIG distinction and where we tend to veer off the road from a person who is drug dependent and one who is addicted. However, the line is so fine and fuzzy that it is often difficult for even the most seasoned professionals to hand down a solid verdict. This is what is so dangerous about this argument.

Yes, the heroin addict generally knows the risks involved when consenting to that first fix. The benzo addict usually does not. Part of the attraction of doing a line of cocaine is the rush of euphoria that comes afterwards. Most benzo addicts are simply following their physician's instructions and are single-mindedly interested in keeping the symptoms of anxiety or insomnia at bay. There are exceptions to this and the distinction between addiction and dependency really comes down to behavior.

Addiction may or may not include the physical component of dependency but it most certainly has everything to do with the reward centers in your brain. We have discussed "How Benzos Work" already and will go through that again soon, but the fact that your brain chemistry has been altered to the point that it's not going to produce the required number of receptors without the drug, gives solid evidence for changes in behavior to make sure that you get that drug into your system on a regular basis. Addiction is characterized by such behaviors as taking more of the medication than prescribed, continuing to use the substances despite negative consequences, compulsive drug seeking behavior or strong focus on the drug and its effects, and craving of the drug even when there are no symptoms to be treated.

It has been argued that drug abuse and drug dependency simply lie at different ends of the same disease process. I agree with this wholeheartedly. While I think that some with a straight dependency can detox and move forward with their lives, never looking back or worrying about those nasty drugs again, it's rare and a scary prospect. It's scary because the addict, reading this, will ALWAYS convince themselves that they are that person. This was once me and it only brought me several more years of pain. The fact of the matter is that, if you have become "dependent" on benzos, why take the chance? Let's call it what it is and move on.

1.5 million Xanax addicts are produced (in the U.S.) each year. - John Steinberg, Medical Director of the Chemical Dependency Program, Greater Baltimore Medical Center

Xanax®
Alprazolam
20mg
PSYCHIATRIC HELP 5¢
THE DOCTOR IS IN

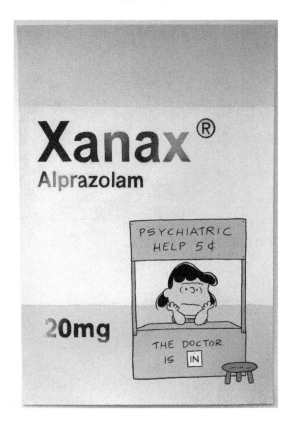

Short Term Use Only

Klonopin - more deadly than coke – Stevie Nicks

Story:

Karen was prescribed Valium by her doctor after a car accident. She had sprained her neck and had a very bad concussion. The physician told her to take 10mg every day to help her muscles relax and heal. She didn't tell Karen that she could become extremely physically dependant after only 28 days. When she went back and told her the weird symptoms she was experiencing, she was told that it was interdose withdrawal and that she should be on a longer acting med.. Klonopin .5 mg 2x a day. With the concussion she couldn't focus, or read well or do anything really except sleep. So she trusted her. she took the meds. Six months later, Karen decided she wanted to taper off after learning everything she could once she could finally read again. So she told the physician she wanted to taper, and she was given a six week taper plan. After two days of his "taper plan" she was hallucinating, vomiting, my skin was crawling, nightmares etc. She has since been abandoned completely by her physician and has to drive 45 minutes to an emergency psych clinic to get her prescription.

What physicians rarely explain to patients as they hand them that first prescription for a benzodiazepine is that these drugs are highly addictive and are recommended only for short-term use. In fact, it has been shown that addiction to benzos can take place in as little as two to four weeks. Sounds like heroin, right? It would be similar if not for the fact that heroin is much easier to get off of than a benzo. The reason that benzodiazepines are so addictive lies in the reward center of the brain that is influenced by the drug.

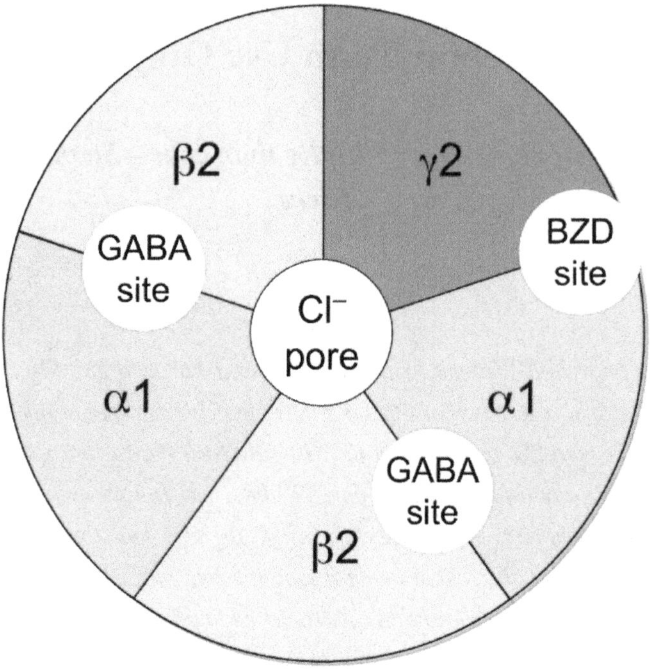

According to Swiss medical researcher, Dr. Christian Luscher, who studies neurobiological pathways to drug addiction, it's all about a certain type of GABA receptor (alpha-1). Dr. Lüscher and colleagues have now demonstrated that benzodiazepines weaken the influence of a group of cells, called inhibitory interneurons, in the brain's ventral tegmental area (VTA). These neurons normally help prevent excessive dopamine levels by downregulating the firing rates of dopamine-producing neurons. Two negatives make a positive, so when benzodiazepines limit the interneurons' restraining influence, the dopamine-producing neurons release more dopamine.

It has long been known that addictive drugs cause long-lasting changes in the reward system of the brain. In this case, there is the migration of certain AMPA receptors from the interior to the surface of the dopamine-producing neurons. Dr. Luscher has shown that benzodiazepines induce AMPA receptor migration via the alpha-1

GABA receptors. Once this happens, the result is addiction that manifests a variety of behaviors and symptoms that aren't pretty.

Signs and Symptoms of Benzo Addiction

When you're an addict, you can go without feeling anything except drunk or stoned or hungry. Still, when you compare this to other feelings, to sadness, anger, fear, worry, despair, and depression, well, an addiction no longer looks so bad. It looks like a very viable option.
- Chuck Palahniuk, Choke

Whether using illicitly (illegally) or not, benzo addiction can creep up fast and, once it's there, the situation can be baffling for those caught in it. Of course, the main effects of benzo abuse are tolerance and addiction. However, there are other symptoms that will show up as well. A person may appear perpetually drowsy and sleepy, lack coordination, or be hostile and irritable. He or she may have vivid and disturbing dreams and may have a poor memory or complete amnesia of some events. Persons using benzos to excess will often not manifest anxiety even if that reaction might be normal for a situation, i.e. - your house is on fire.

Here are some other signs and symptoms of addiction:

1. A strong desire or sense of compulsion to take the substance.
2. Impaired capacity to control substance-taking behavior in terms of onset, termination or level of use, as evidenced by: the substance being often taken in larger amounts or over a longer period than intended, or any unsuccessful effort or persistent desire to cut down or control substance use.

3. A physiological withdrawal state when substance use is reduced or ceased, as evidenced by the characteristic withdrawal syndrome for the substance, or use of the same (or closely related) substance with the intention of relieving or avoiding withdrawal symptoms.

4. Evidence of tolerance to the effects of the substance, such that there is a need for markedly increased amounts of the substance to achieve intoxication or desired effect, or that there is a markedly diminished effect with continued use of the same amount of the substance.

5. Preoccupation with substance use, as manifested by: important alternative pleasures or interests being given up or reduced because of substance use; or a great deal of time being spent in activities necessary to obtain the substance, take the substance, or recover from its effects.

6. Persisting with substance use despite clear evidence of harmful consequences, as evidenced by continued use when the person was actually aware of, or could be expected to have been aware of the nature and extent of harm.

In essence, if you have been on benzos for a prolonged period of time, have developed a tolerance requiring increased dosages, have an inability to cope without the drugs, or have suffered any negative consequences (family, work, financial, emotional) as a result of using them, you have entered addiction territory. This is a scary prospect for many, and particularly for those who arrived at this point via a legitimate physician's prescription and a lot of trust. Regardless of how you got here, there is hope and we're going to make the assumption that you are looking to break free based upon your purchase of this book. There is still much to learn about benzos before we get there, though.

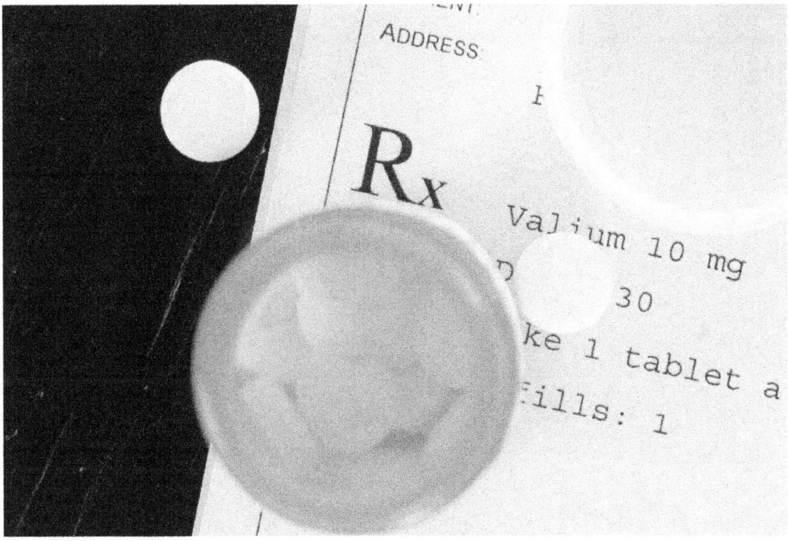
ADDRESS:
Rx
Valium 10 mg
30

Benzo Overdose Considerations

And if you take more of those, you will get an overdose
No more running for the shelter of a mother's little helper
They just helped you on your way, through your busy dying day - Keith Richards, Mick Jagger

---

If you find that you've become addicted to benzos, don't stop taking them. This is one of the most dangerous things that you can do. I'm going to state this over and over again to make sure that the point gets across. It's commonly believed that you can't overdose on benzodiazepines alone. Some will debate this because, if you are elderly or have some underlying serious health or mental conditions, it is a likely possibility that you can put yourself in serious physical jeopardy with a massive dose of benzos.

Barring that, the most common instances of benzo overdoses happen when they are taken in combination with other substances. This is very serious. Every 19 minutes in this country, someone dies of a prescription drug related overdose covering all categories of drugs; 36 percent of these overdoses involve prescription opiates. Concurrently, benzodiazepines have increasingly become part of a deadly combination with opiates that can seriously depress respiratory and heart function to a point where death is the all-too-common final outcome.

Benzodiazepines have additive effects with other CNS depressants, including other hypnotics, sedative antidepressants, neuroleptics, anticonvulsants, sedative antihistamines, and alcohol. The combined disinhibitory effects of alcohol and benzodiazepines may also be additive and contribute to aggressive behavior. According to Dr. Michael Kelley, the medical director of the behavioral department at St. Mary's Regional Medical Center in Lewiston, Maine, these drugs actually "potentiate each other — they make each other stronger. And so one plus one doesn't equal two; it equals three or four." Patients prescribed benzodiazepines should be warned of these interactions.

Tramadol (Ultram) has long been thought to be a safe pain management alternative to prescription opiates (it's not). Not only are they just as addictive as any other opiate, like Vicodin or heroin, used in combination with benzos, they can be deadly. Opioids and benzos work differently in the body, but as CNS depressants they compound the effects of one another. All CNS depressants are cross-tolerant with one another meaning that developing a tolerance for one will result in a tolerance for another. A person who has used benzos for any length of time will find that Tramadol is not as effective as expected, and the patient is likely to take larger than recommended doses of the drug. Taking larger doses increases the risk of overdose, particularly when CNS depressants are combined. Benzodiazepine use can increase the lethality of Tramadol, and, while benzos alone do not usually produce fatal overdose, they can when used in conjunction with an opioid. The combined sedative effects of Tramadol and benzos are enough to cause death from depressed breathing.

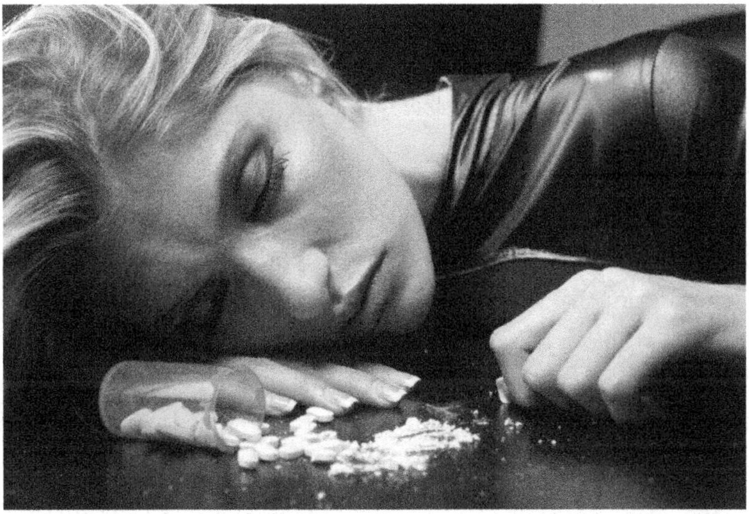

Another drug combination that is both popular and deadly is known to some as "The Holy Trinity". This involves the combination of a benzo, an opiate, and carisoprodol (Soma). The three have some overlapping side effects in terms of drowsiness, respiratory depression, confusion, tremors, and seizure risk. When combined, these drugs are synergistic in causing respiratory depression and could collectively result in death.

Story:

Pete Jackson attended his brother-in-law's funeral along with his daughter, Emily, six years ago. He never dreamed it would be the last day of his daughter's life. "It's so tragic, just not something you would never, ever expect," said Pete Jackson.

Instead of going home to the Chicago suburb of Arlington Heights after the funeral, Emily Jackson, 18, spent the night with her cousins. That night, she made a deadly decision. She took an Oxycontin -- a single prescription pill -- that her cousin offered to her while drinking. She went to sleep that night and never woke up. She died of respiratory depression -- she simply stopped breathing.

The Oxycontin that Emily took belonged to her uncle, who had died of cancer. While taking one pill and dying is rare, dying accidentally after using painkillers in combination with other drugs or alcohol is common.

When benzodiazepines are abused with other drugs, the effect can be coma or death. Hundreds of thousands of people go to US emergency rooms each year for problems with benzodiazepine abuse. Hospital emergency room visits for benzodiazepine abuse now dwarf those for illegal street drugs by a more than a three-to-one margin. This trend has been increasing for at least the last five years. In 2006, the U.S. government's Substance Abuse and Mental Health Services Administration (SAMSHA) published data showing that prescription drugs that year were the number two reason for ER admissions to hospitals for drug abuse, slightly behind illicit substances like heroin and cocaine. According to data from SAMSHA, the instances of benzo and narcotic pain reliever admissions increased 569.7% in the 10 years from 2000 to 2010.

Figure 1. Estimated number of emergency department (ED) visits involving benzodiazepines alone or in combination with opioids or alcohol,* by year and drug combination (patients aged 12 and older): 2005 to 2011

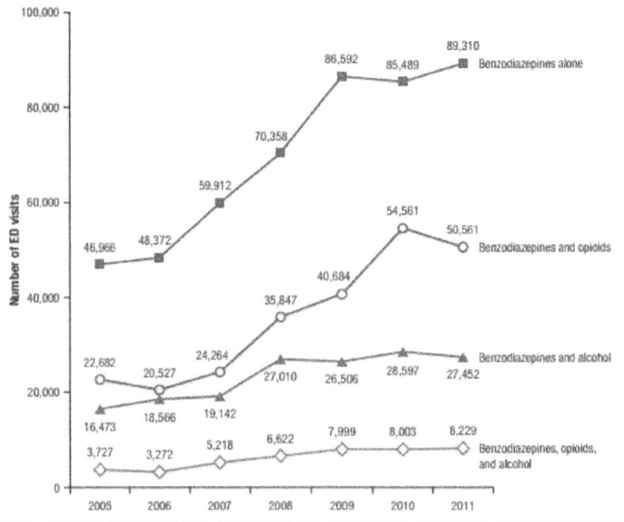

* No other drugs were involved.

Source: 2005 to 2011 SAMHSA Drug Abuse Warning Network (DAWN).

Special Considerations with Benzo Addiction

While there isn't an addiction out there without its quirks and unique qualities about it, benzodiazepine addiction seems to have more than most. There are a lot of things to be aware of and understand if you have become dependent upon benzos. These are the types of things that we are going to cover in this section.

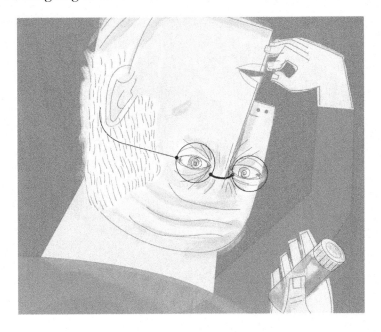

Long-term Use of Benzos Ignores Underlying Issues

Doctors have throughout time made fortunes on killing their patients with their cures. The difference in psychiatry is that it is the death of the soul. - R.D. Laing, MD

Whether it be anxiety, depression, or a seizure disorder, benzodiazepines are miracle drugs to treat these symptoms and practically make them vanish in very short order. What isn't often explained to the patient, however, is that they do not actually "cure" these disorders and that the drugs are only designed to be taken on a short-term basis. Unless something is done to treat the underlying issue, little progress has been made other than to give the patient some short-term relief disguised as hope for a long-term cure. These little pills will never accomplish that.

I'm sure there are those who will wish to send me hate mail and differing opinions on this matter. Please do if it makes you feel better but, the fact of the matter is that, prescribing these meds for an issue is like dropping one of those bouncy balls from some unknown, random, height. Once it hits the ground and makes its way back into the sky, you'll understand.

The Rebound Effect

Sometimes I say the medication is even tougher than the illness. - Sanya Richards-Ross

The bounce, or rebound effect, with benzos is a real thing and the most obscene case of irony should you be taking these for such things as anxiety or insomnia. In essence, the symptoms that you started taking the drugs for in the first place actually manifest in a much more pronounced fashion. Say you were taking Xanax for Generalized Anxiety Disorder (GAD). After awhile (probably not too long), you begin to feel as if you are coming unglued around the time that your dose of Xanax begins to wear off. You become convinced that you must have a very severe anxiety disorder because of this, maybe even one requiring a higher dose of the medication to treat properly.

Believe it or not, approximately 70% of patients who take benzos experience rebound symptoms that are worse than those that they had before they started taking the medication in the first place. Sometimes these occur after benzos have been discontinued, but many times this is happening while the patient is still taking the benzos. Either a shorter-acting benzo is causing rebound insomnia (or anxiety) in the night or early morning, or there could be issues with tolerance.

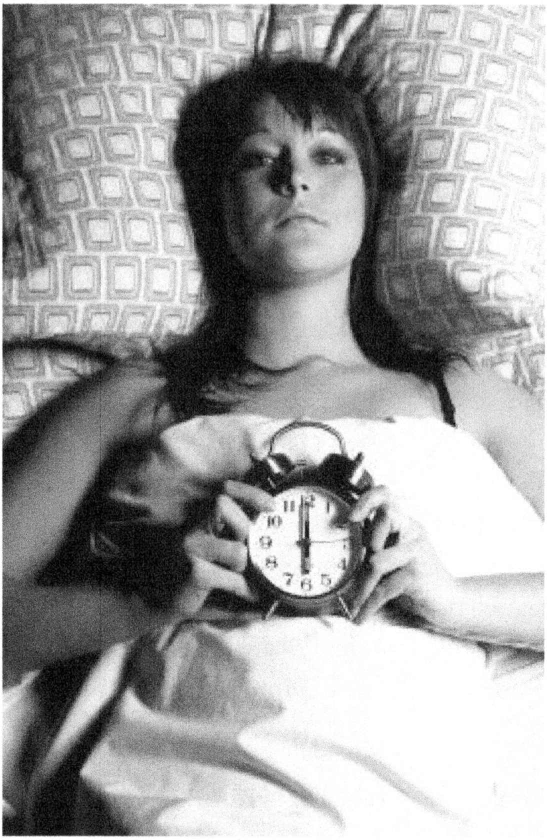

Tolerance and Tolerance Withdrawal

The only difference between a drug addict and the rest of society is the drug. - Krivanek

Again, because these are only to be taken short-term, this shouldn't be an issue. But we all know that this isn't what has been happening for the past fifty years so those who have been on benzos for any period of time are going to need more of the drug to get the same, or desired, effect. This is called tolerance. Even those who have been on a steady dosage for years will eventually reach a point where the drugs aren't working for them anymore. Their body and brain have adapted to the drug and are asking for more. When it doesn't receive it, it starts to go into what is called "tolerance withdrawal" and the patient gets very sick.

I know for a fact now that this is what happened to my 73 year old mother, who was on Ativan for many years and then was suddenly sick for over 3 months. No one could figure out what was wrong with her until she went to a new primary care physician who took her off of the benzos, and I had to rush her to the emergency room. The cunning thing about these withdrawal symptoms is that they are often similar or identical to the symptoms for which the patient was taking the medication in the first place. When these symptoms occur, the choice is there: Either find a way to get off of these things once and for all or find a way to continue the madness.

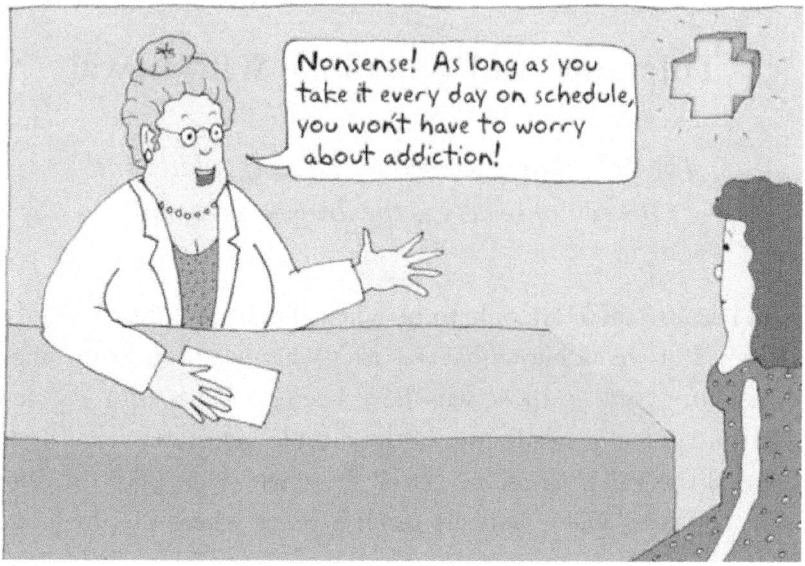
Nonsense! As long as you take it every day on schedule, you won't have to worry about addiction!

Drugs Create a New "Normal"

You can tranquilize your mind
So go running for the shelter of a mother's little helper
And four help you through the night, help to minimize your plight
Doctor please, some more of these
Outside the door, she took four more
What a drag it is getting old - Keith Richards, Mick Jagger

Let's get one thing straight. A perpetual state of calm and relaxation, sedation even, is not "normal". Normal people deal with anxious moments, fear, joy, intimacy, and a myriad of other elements in the human experience that drugs make simply impossible. When your sole aim in life is to be free of any sort of anxiety, worry, or panic, this is no longer living. Instead, it is escaping and some would argue that it is well on the way to dying.

I can so relate to this because it was me for a long time. In the beginning, drugs gave me the relief that I was looking for from the stresses of everyday life - and my life wasn't that bad! In the end, I couldn't feel anything anymore and felt trapped in a deep, dark hole. If this is you, it doesn't mean that you're a bad person, just a lost one. Being uncomfortable at times is a part of life and crawling out of that deep, dark hole is completely possible. Keep reading.

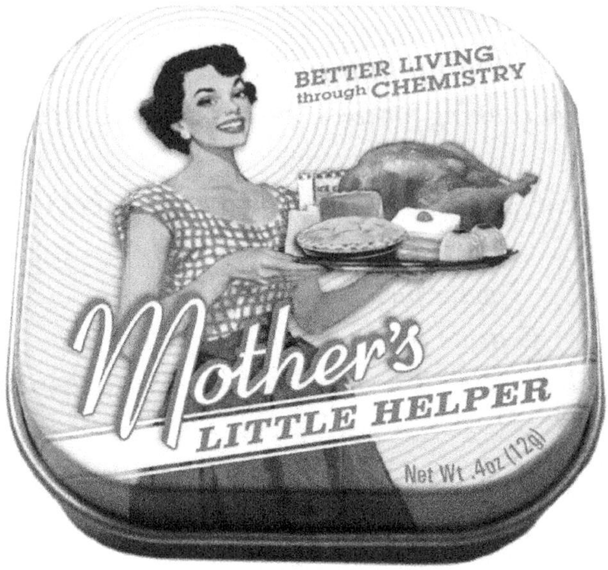
BETTER LIVING
through CHEMISTRY
Mother's
LITTLE HELPER
Net Wt .4oz (12g)

Drugs Create an Obsession with Self

The worst thing about addiction is that you spend all day thinking about how to stop thinking about it. - James Yager

I really didn't understand until I got clean and sober how self-absorbed and self-obsessed I was while using drugs. I know that we all think that we are "different" or unique and therein lies part of the problem. Because benzodiazepines themselves are psychotropic drugs, this brings this issue to an entirely new level. For most, the onset of use of these drugs wasn't for a chronic pain issue or a social reason, although there are exceptions. For most, it was to change the way you feel at the deepest level.

This use of a drug specifically to change the way you feel has the added effect of re-focusing the patient on exactly that - 24/7. What a concept. The person using benzos is now focused more inward than ever before and becomes even more obsessed with how they are feeling at any given moment. This is no way to live and certainly no way to live happily. Experiencing life on life's terms requires the interaction and participation of others and the self-centered drug addict is quite incapable of doing this.

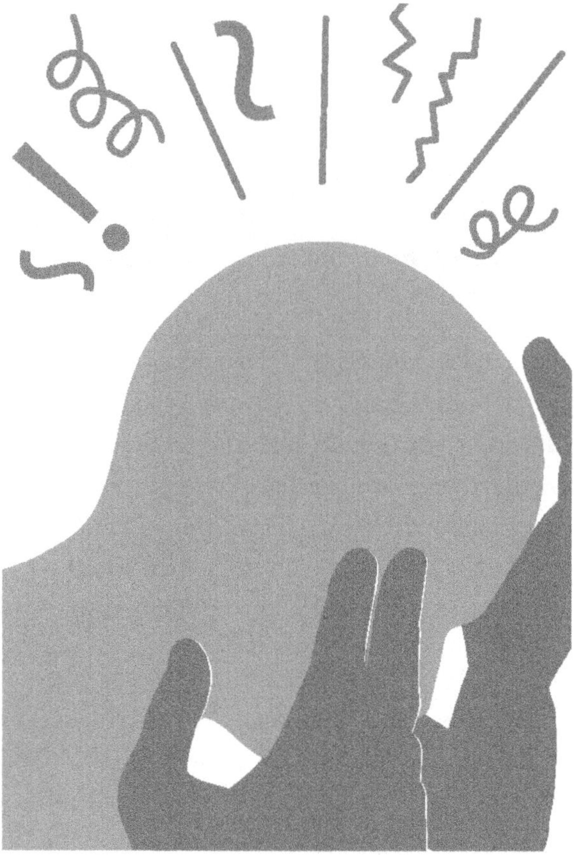

Perpetual State of Impairment

Drugs are a bet with your mind. — Jim Morrison

Benzos, whether taken once or multiple times a day, will eventually put the user in a perpetual state of impairment. They can make a person appear intoxicated by causing slurred speech, forgetfulness, and sometimes silly behavior. Some people are completely uninhibited or have different personalities when using benzos.

Regardless, because of the their effects, it is not recommended that one drive or operate machinery after taking benzos. Consistent with loss of visuospatial ability and speed of processing, it was found that benzodiazepine use was associated with driving problems like deviation from one's lane. Those tested the day after taking benzodiazepines showed a similar loss of driving skills similar to a blood alcohol concentration of .05 to .10 (the federally mandated legal limit is .08).

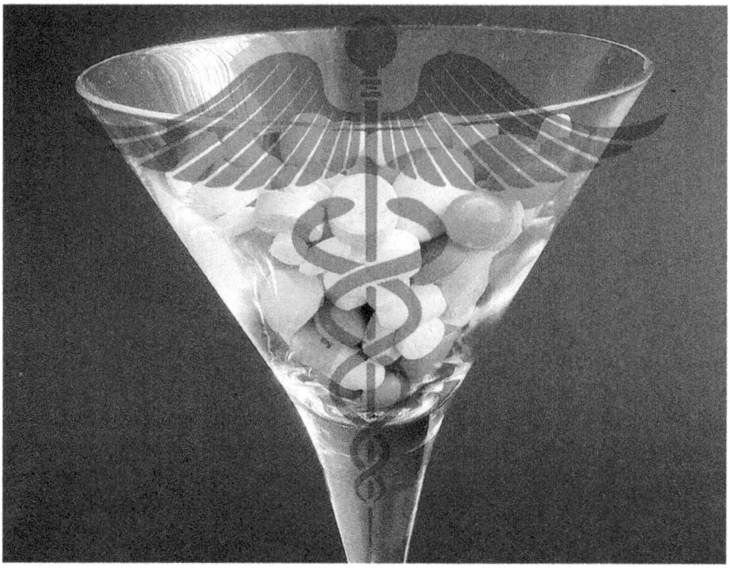

Also, a woman who takes benzodiazepines during pregnancy risks having her baby develop a cleft in the mouth, withdrawal symptoms and floppy infant syndrome, a condition in which the baby lacks muscle tone and does not develop normally. There is also risk of early miscarriage.

Cross Addictions Often Develop

In the course of history many more people have died for their drink and their dope than have died for their religion or their country. - Aldous Huxley

---

I don't know about you but, when I was drinking and using drugs, I became convinced that I could not function on a day-to-day basis without taking something - anything. If one thing was removed or I was unable to obtain my drug of choice, I would take whatever I could get. If I liked the new substance enough, I would also become addicted to that one. This is called cross addiction and it is more common than many think.

Because benzos operate on the same receptors in the brain as alcohol, barbiturates, and opiates, it's pretty easy to see how cross addiction can happen. This doesn't mean that you can substitute something else for benzos and not suffer withdrawal symptoms. Unfortunately, that isn't the case at all. However, it is very common to combine these drugs and, as we discussed in the last section, they can be very dangerous combinations.

Story:

The devastation began for Steve Rummler when he got a prescription for nerve pain radiating through his leg and back. It started when he was 28. For the next nine years, the Minneapolis man endured the pain. It was not until 2005, when Rummler was 37, that a doctor prescribed hydrocodone to address his pain, along with clonazepam, a benzodiazepine and anti-anxiety medication, to relieve his injury-related anxiety.

Family members said it was the first time in nearly a decade Rummler felt relief from the life-altering pain he endured. But that relief was short-lived. In a journal entry, Rummler said of the drugs, "At first they were a lifeline. Now they are a noose around my neck."

By 2009, Rummler had sunk into dependence and, eventually, into addiction. At the advice of his family, he enrolled in two addiction treatment programs and seemingly had a handle on his addiction. But in July of 2011, just 45 days after completing the final stage of his rehabilitation, Rummler relapsed and died at 43.

Rummler still had outstanding prescriptions for hydrocodone and clonazepam at the time of his death, and empty prescription bottles were in his house when the police arrived. His official cause of death was mixed drug toxicity caused by opiates and benzodiazepines.

Long Term Health Issues

For years, most doctors have assumed that benzodiazepines must have worked because patients kept taking them.....thus dependence has been reinforced – as has the belief that these drugs can go on working for years. - Charles Medawar Social Audit

---

So far, the most serious long term health concern that anyone should have with regards to benzodiazepines is addiction. Aside from that, there are other health concerns that anyone who takes these drugs needs to be aware of.

In 2005, a study was published in the Journal of Clinical Psychology that stated that not only did the use of benzodiazepines interfere with visuospatial ability, speed of processing thoughts and perceptions and the ability to absorb verbal lessons, but also after a person withdrew from benzodiazepine use, these abilities did not fully return. Those who used benzodiazepines over a longer period of time were more impaired. It is interesting to note that while prescribing instructions specifically state that benzodiazepines should not be given for a long term, the participants in this study had been taking this type of drug for an average of nine years.

Even more disturbing, a study published in the British Medical Journal in 2014 by a team of researchers from France and Canada has linked benzodiazepine use to an increased risk of being diagnosed with Alzheimer's Disease. Based on the study, the greater a person's cumulative dose of benzos, the higher his or her risk of Alzheimer's. While this is only one study, it's definitely worth taking note of.

According to their findings, taking the drug for three to six months raised the risk of developing Alzheimer's by 32%, and taking it for more than six months boosted the risk by 84%. The type of drug taken also mattered. People who were on a long-acting benzodiazepine like diazepam (Valium) and flurazepam (Dalmane) were at greater risk than those on a short-acting one like triazolam (Halcion), lorazepam (Ativan), alprazolam (Xanax), and temazepam (Restoril). The researchers acknowledge that the use of benzodiazepines could be just a signal that people are trying to cope with anxiety and sleep disruption—two common symptoms of early Alzheimer's disease. If that's true, their use of a benzodiazepine may not be a factor in causing dementia but an indication it is already in progress.

Story:

Susan took care of her parents in their home until their deaths in 2012. Both parents took most all of the above-listed drugs listed in the study for years (from the 1970s to 2012). As they aged, they were prescribed more and more of increasing doses of said drugs. Both were diagnosed with Alzheimer's dementia and both died from the effects of Alzheimer's dementia. Their care went from daily small things to continual round-the-clock care and finally hospice. Having extensively studied her family history for over 30 years, Susan cannot find one biological relative who had any evidence of Alzheimer's dementia on either her father or mother's side of the family. At one point, her parents' addiction to this drug was so bad, they required hospitalization in a psychiatric ward, trying withdrawal schedules, etc., and the family members both fighting this all the way, seeing the handwriting on the wall of what was to come, and yet this drug was prescribed like water. In the end, both of their deaths were directly linked to Alzheimer dementia with the textbook symptoms.

Finally, if you or your loved are over the age of 65 and have been taking benzodiazepines for any length of time, there are other reasons to avoid them if you aren't already convinced. In 2012 the American Geriatrics Society added benzodiazepines to their list (called the BEERs List) of inappropriate medications for treating insomnia, agitation, or delirium. That decision was made primarily because common side-effects of benzodiazepines - confusion and clouded thinking - often have disastrous consequences, including falls, fractures, and auto accidents. Even short-acting benzodiazepines pack a bigger punch in older people. As the body's metabolism slows with age, drugs take longer to clear. And because benzodiazepines are stored in body fat, they can continue to produce effects days after people stop taking them.

Withdrawal from Benzos

We cannot, in a moment, get rid of habits of a lifetime. - Mahatma Gandhi

---

First and foremost, what is "detox" as it relates to withdrawal? A "toxin" is anything that impedes normal functions of the body, or causes stagnation, congestion or dis-ease. What keeps things from being toxic? The circulatory, lymph system, colon, liver, urinary system, etc. 'Blockage' of any of these systems - for example, by making them work too hard, or overloading them - can ultimately result in toxins accumulating in the body. "Detoxification" or 'detox' refers to the period of time it takes for the 'active' toxins to leave the body -- as little as a week or as long as several months.

Benzodiazepine withdrawal is unlike any other drug because of its danger, intensity and duration. Oftentimes, people have no idea that they've become dependent upon these drugs until they try to go off of them and become violently ill, many times with life-threatening consequences. Whether withdrawal sets in as a result of stopping the medication or due to a tolerance issue that has built up, the symptoms are quite unpleasant and can include extreme anxiety, paranoia, and agoraphobia. A longer list of benzo withdrawal symptoms is as follows:

- Perceptual distortions
- Paraesthesia, defined as abnormal skin sensations such as tingling, tickling, itching or burning
- Difficult walking
- Anxiety
- Tension
- Agitation

- Restlessness
- Sleep disturbance/insomnia
- Feelings of unreality
- Extreme dysphoria (depression, unease, dissatisfaction with life)
- Depersonalization (state in which a person feels that their feelings or thoughts belong to someone other than himself/herself; loss of sense of personal identity)
- Feelings of persecution
- Paranoid thoughts
- Pain/headache
- Seizures
- Depression
- Psychosis
- Confusional states
- Fits

Because the risk of seizures is there with benzo withdrawal, it is crucial that you NEVER stop taking them altogether or try to detox "cold turkey" from them. This is highly dangerous and has resulted in death. As benzodiazepine detox can be drawn out, complicated, and quite uncomfortable, it is generally recommended that you take it slow with a tapered detox at home or check yourself into a medical detox facility if your situation warrants.

It's also important to note that everyone's body and brain react differently. Therefore, what is a terrible detox for one person may not be anything at all to someone else. Frankly, I didn't have a lot of trouble coming off of benzos 14 years ago, but I also didn't know any better. I had been taking them for years along with other drugs and pretty much stopped everything at once.

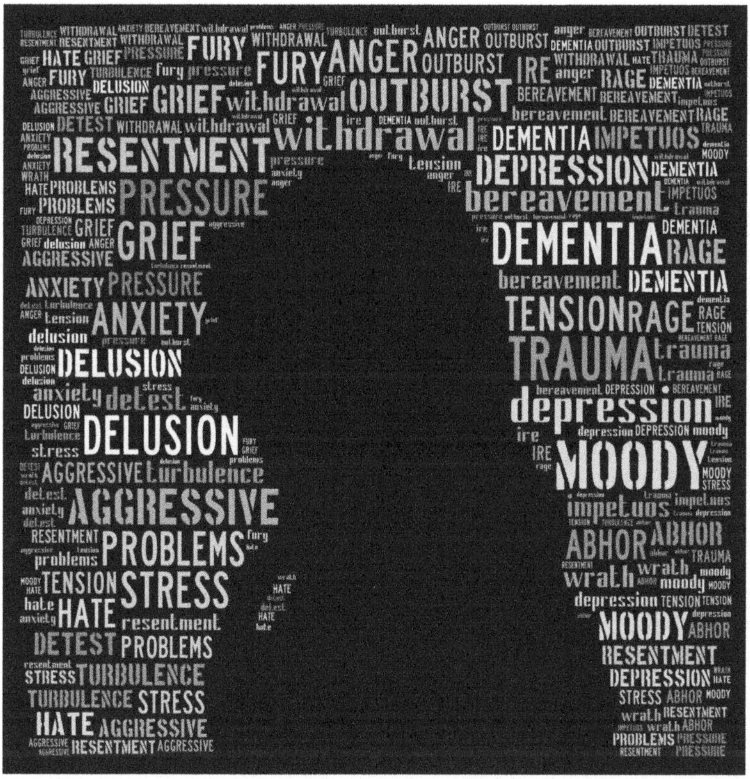

According to Professor C Heather Ashton, one of the world's authorities on this subject, 30%-40% of patients who have used regular therapeutic doses of benzodiazepines for more than a few months are at risk of experiencing withdrawal symptoms. However, those who have abused the drugs at high levels are almost certain to experience symptoms. Certain potent, rapidly metabolized benzodiazepines (alprazolam, triazolam, lorazepam) have been associated with more severe and acute withdrawal symptoms. Dosage (within the therapeutic range) and duration of benzodiazepine use (above 6 to 12 months) do not appear to affect the incidence or severity of withdrawal, but anxious and passive-dependent personality types and alcohol-dependent subjects may be especially vulnerable.

Now that we've made it completely ambiguous, there is still a choice to be made. As far as getting off of benzos is concerned, there are probably more wrong ways to get off of these drugs than right ways. As such, we are going to take a close look at all of your options including: detox situations to avoid, a medical detox facility, the home detox with tapering, and the various tapering options available. There is a lot to take in and it's important to remember that not all options are recommended for everyone and that everyone's experiences with these WILL vary.

How NOT to Detox From Benzos

Imagine trying to live without air. Now imagine something worse. — Amy Reed, Clean

Cold Turkey Detox

I don't think that we could possibly say it enough times in this book - Don't simply stop taking your benzodiazepines! Even if you have heard of others doing this with success, it is never worth the risk. Stopping benzos cold turkey puts you at risk for seizures, psychosis and possibly death. The following severity of symptoms could necessitate that you simply resume benzo use and some even put off a proper withdrawal as a result.

Story:

I started taking Xanax about 5 years ago to help me sleep at first and also to help me with my anxiety/panic attacks that I started having due to work/medical issues/IBS issues. It worked very well for me at around .5mg per day at bedtime, however, I ended up with a really awful GP doc who ultimately upped my dosage all the way to 8.0mg per day. I was not told the severe ramifications of stopping this medication "cold turkey" and I actually ran out while we were out of town for 11 days and I honestly thought I would die! What is even more interesting is that I finally realized, because I ran out early and had no choice but to start researching this, that I was becoming an agoraphobic and had worsening symptoms of anxiety as the dosages increased, but my doc didn't tell me any of this. I was ALWAYS hearing the warnings about being on pain medication and how BAD the withdrawal and side effects were, but Xanax seemed to be the "Mom's Best Friend" for most of my friends, to just take the edge off and allow us to better cope with work/life balance. NO dice my friends! Do NOT go off of this medication without educating yourself about the severe ramifications of it because you MAY think that you are going to die, you will suffer from things that NOBODY has EVER warned you about and it is the worst thing I've ever had to go through in my life. Absolutely do your research before you go off of this medication!

Rapid Benzo Detox (RBD)

There are a (very) few benzo detox centers that will claim to get your system free of benzodiazepines within a matter of days. These procedures are very expensive, not proven, and often lead to severe protracted withdrawal symptoms, which we discuss later in the next section. If a detox center tells you that they are going to use "Flumazenil", do your due diligence before agreeing to something like this as results have not been consistent or encouraging.

Anonymous story:

It didn't work for me. The cost was $5,650. Dr. X and his staff were extremely nice. There were two others there that it worked for. I'm sure after they left they went through withdrawal??? Dr. X does say that. He does not stuff you with meds like people say that haven't been there. He gives you a med for 7 days to prevent seizures. Your there all day with him the first day being monitored and the days after you come to see him every day for the consecutive days of treatment, even on Saturdays and Sundays. After the treatment is done he likes to see you almost weekly after that. He does care about you. He wants you off of the drugs! It did feel like a cold turkey for me minus the physical withdrawals. He says it works for 8 out of 10 people. I had to reinstate and I felt insane.

Going to Detox

I am dying with the aid of too many doctors. - Alexander the Great

Because benzodiazepine detox is considered to be so dangerous, many people just assume that they need to be rushed to the nearest emergency room or medical detox center in order to be "removed" from these drugs. I did and it's actually a dangerous misconception due to the nature of the drug and the time that it takes to detox from it. Most, nearly all, detox facilities are not set up to properly manage the detox of a patient that should take months (or longer) if done properly. You are going to find the marketing departments of various treatment centers telling you differently. Don't be swayed. Unless you meet some specific criteria, this one probably shouldn't be top on your list.

So, why would you go to a medical detox facility for benzo detox? Several reasons you will need to consider this one:

- If benzos were taken in combination with other drugs, such as opiates, or alcohol and an in-patient setting is needed to manage detox from multiple substances.

- If there are co-occurring medical or psychiatric issues that are going to make a home detox more difficult or dangerous. This could include such things as pulmonary disease, heart conditions, or other psychiatric issues. A lot of times, alcohol and drugs are used to ease or relieve the symptoms of a psychiatric disorder. When the use stops, the original psychiatric symptoms that were suppressed and acute withdrawal can come forth simultaneously and this needs to be managed in a controlled, professional setting. You will need to enlist your physician's help in making these decisions.

- You either lack the self-discipline or don't have the support of others who can help manage your taper and act as a caretaker if needed.

These are all very real concerns and, if any of them could apply to you, please discuss them with your loved ones and your physician before making your choice. Otherwise, most people who detox from benzos do so over an extended period of time and do it at home.

Detoxing from Benzos at Home

Before you can break out of prison, you must realize you are locked up. - unknown

Home Detox Considerations

The type of withdrawals, their intensity, the duration, and the preparations necessary for detox are going to depend entirely on the type of drug being abused as well as the scale of abuse. Certain drugs most definitely have a more intense and prolonged detoxification period, and some can even be dangerous or life-threatening. There are many things to consider before undertaking a home detox so that you are successful, comfortable and safe.

Why Are You Stopping?

Don't gloss over this - it's huge. In fact, it's a whole other book but unless you have some understanding of why you are doing this, this is going to be wasted time (pun intended). While it's ok to want to stop taking these drugs for other people, you also have to want to stop doing so for your own sake. If legal, financial, work and family consequences are piling up as a result of your addiction, how does this make you feel? If these things are making you tired of using these drugs, you're probably in the right place.

If you are still not sure about this, list out the positive and negative aspects of your drug use. Even if you consider yourself one of those "accidental addicts", it won't hurt you to play along. Seriously, get out a piece of paper and a pen. What are these things bringing to your life?

Be honest, this list is only for your benefit and doesn't need to be shared with anyone else. For many, in the beginning, drugs made them feel good or took away some sort of pain, either physical or emotional. However, that is just a "chased" feeling in the end and it doesn't work anymore. In the end, most people can see that drugs, when used to excess (either in quantity or for too long), actually took them away from the social scene, left them isolated, were damaging their health, hurt family and friends, were illegal or caused them to do things that were illegal, diminished their self-image and had many more negative aspects than positive. Be courageous and make your list before you go any further.

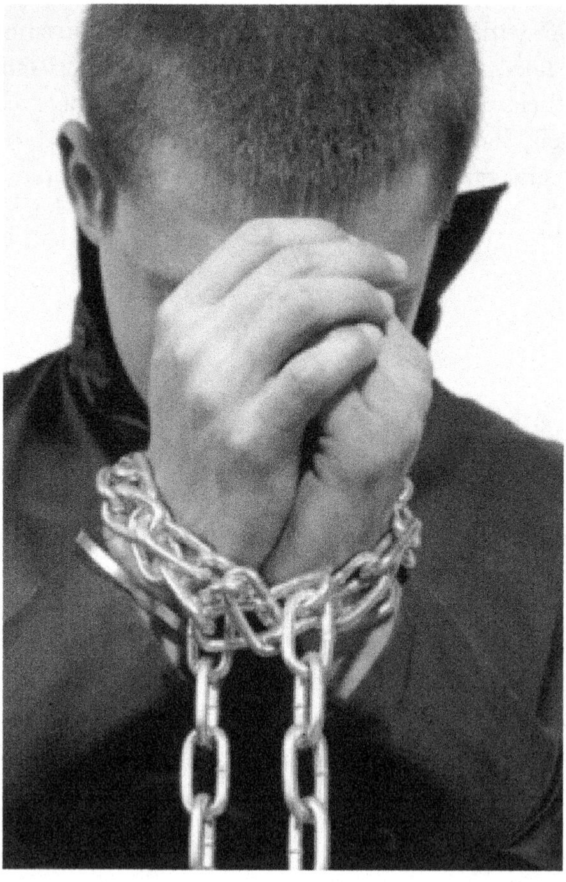

What Drugs Are You Using?

Stopping the addictive use of any substance is going to have some affects; it doesn't matter if it's over-the-counter Benadryl or Heroin. However, there is a huge difference in the type of physical and psychological withdrawal that will occur when you stop taking them and the duration of those symptoms. Many addicts don't take just one thing either. They may take opiates during the day and Benzos at night to sleep. Or they may drink during the day and take sedatives at night. So, make a list of all of the drugs (including alcohol) that you are taking on a daily basis and the quantities. Again, be honest here. And, again, this isn't a mental list - find that pen! This is your detox and you are going to be running the show (mostly). If you want to be successful, you can't downplay or gloss over anything.

There is ongoing debate as to whether withdrawal from certain drugs is classified as "physical" or merely psychological. It's widely agreed that physical symptoms can be expected when you detox from: opiates (heroin, methadone, oxycodone), benzodiazepines (valium, ativan), barbiturates (seconal, fioricet) and alcohol. It was thought for many years that marijuana and amphetamines were not addictive but that you would simply experience mental craving after stopping their use. (This is nothing to shake a stick at, by the way). These notions are actually being re-examined as more studies are done. However, if stopping a substance results in you being unable to concentrate or sleep, chances are there will be some physical consequences. Additionally, cocaine withdrawal is now thought to have a physical component to it as well as the intense psychological craving.

Note: it is not recommended that you just quit using benzos yet keep drinking, smoking marijuana, or taking opiate painkillers on the side. It ALL has to go. If you are addicted to and getting ready to detox from multiple drugs, either consider an inpatient medical detox or take a look at my other book that covers home detox from all of these substances. There are too many for me to list in a book about benzodiazepines. Again, get your list of substances and usage levels done so that you know what you are going to be dealing with and can be prepared if you are going to detox at home.

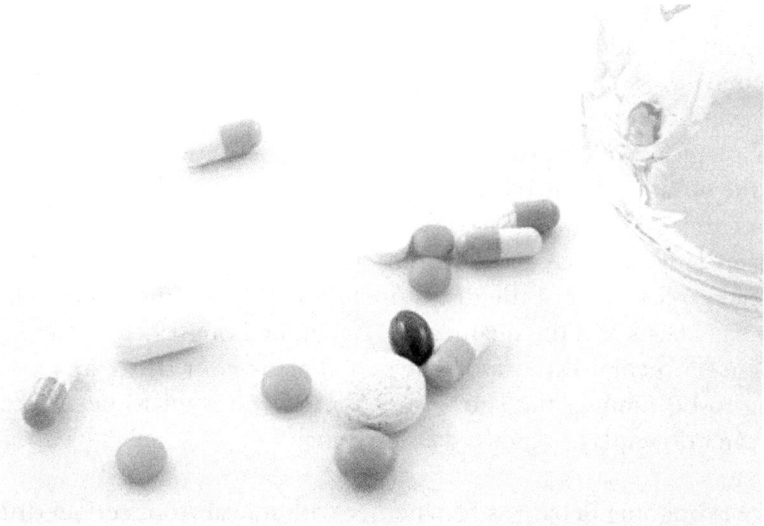

Who is Your Supplier?

Every good drug addict has a supplier and back-up, or ten. Don't wait until after you go through detox to consider this. How were you obtaining your drugs on a regular basis and what is your plan of action with regards to that source(s) in the future? This could very well be the family doctor or your psychiatrist when we are talking about benzos. Depending on the circumstances, and your willingness, you should absolutely try to enlist this professional as an "ally" in your detoxification procedure. All of the recommendations for a home detox will call for a prescription for benzos. So, if you have an understanding physician in your corner, this would be the time to set up an appointment and let them know your plans and your humble request for help. Otherwise, check out the Resources section of the book for some websites that may be able to help you find an understanding and helpful physician for your detox.

If you obtained your drugs illegally, consider that you are going to have to break ties with these contacts. You will need to delete them from your phone, block the numbers, do whatever you need to do. The temptations and cravings will be very strong at times and this is one of the reasons why some self-examination is important before starting the process. Know why you are doing this and be fully committed. Don't give yourself a bunch of "outs" and escape routes if you want to be successful. This is an extremely difficult endeavor to do alone.

Get Some Support

Asking for help does not mean that we are weak or incompetent. It usually indicates an advanced level of honesty and intelligence. - Jim Rohn

For some, the whole idea of doing a home detox means that they want to do this "alone" and have no one know about it. This is both difficult and dangerous. It's difficult because we can be our own worst enemies and because addiction is such a powerful disease that cravings are tough to combat when all alone. It's dangerous because of the physical, and sometimes psychological, component to detox and withdrawal. When not in a medically supervised setting, detox can be scary at times and there may be rare instances where medical intervention is necessary. If you don't have someone that is checking up on you and monitoring your progress, you may not be in the proper state to make that call.

If possible, enlist a family member or friend to help you through the most difficult days of this process. A person who also has alcohol or drug-related problems would not be a good candidate for this role. Your support person's availability to help you and be present for you, ideally, most of the time during the difficult days would be important. Depending on what substance you are withdrawing from, this will vary on which days the symptoms start to how long they last.

A support person can be invaluable in reminding us of why it is that we're doing this in the first place. Believe me, it's easy to forget when the only thing in the forefront of your mind is getting the discomfort to stop in the quickest way possible. If you think that "no one knows" about your problem, you're likely mistaken. It may be worth it to put yourself out there to a trusted friend, family member, or two and experience the relief that comes when you have someone else on your side and rooting for your success. If "everyone knows", there's probably a family member or old friend out there that would love to see you get clean and would be there for you if you asked.

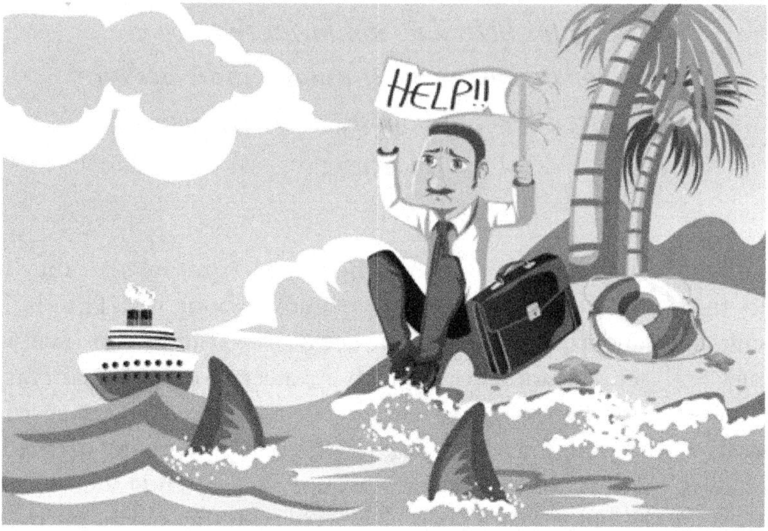

Have a Detox Plan

It's not the load that breaks you down; it's the way you carry it. -Lena Horne

Obviously you've thought about this and are doing some research. These are the sorts of people that put searches in Google and buy books on these things. Good move. Aside from that great first step though, this is a general outline of the plan that you need to put together. Here's the Home Detox Plan:

- Take a look at yourself and why you are stopping (a little self examination exercise)
- Make a List of all of the substances that you are using and quantities
- Call for a Doctor's Appointment
- Clear your Calendar - no big trips or other heavy obligations, although you can continue to work if doing a long tapered detox
- Get some support - Find family or friends that can help you through this
- Put your detox plan together based on your particular substance
- Get things to keep you occupied and entertained when not feeling well - books, movies, etc.
- Begin Detox process
- Keep a detox calendar and diary/journal to track your progress
- Don't use any more drugs or alcohol or switch to something "new".
- Consider a support group afterwards (and even during when you are able to get out).

Beyond Benzos

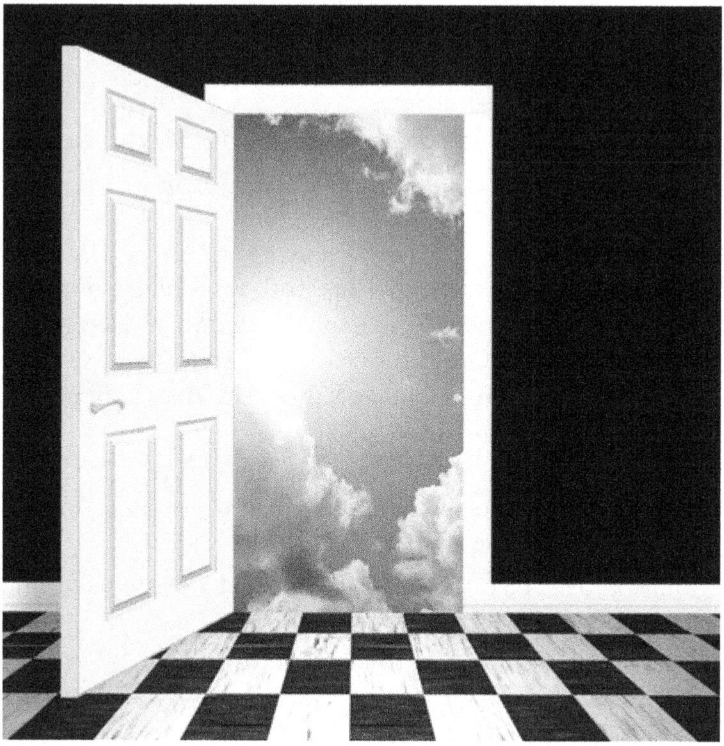

Benzodiazepine Detox and the Importance of Tapering

You cannot just stop takings Benzos "cold turkey". It is entirely too dangerous and can result in severe withdrawal symptoms such as seizures, psychosis and suicide. There are some detox facilities that will do a "cold turkey" detox with the help of a 7 day course of phenobarbitol to ease the symptoms. This is also not recommended because, once that course is completed and the phenobarbitol wears off, the onset of delayed and severe Benzo withdrawals will often kick in and you will be just as miserable as ever. As stated before, a few other detox facilities may use what is called a "flumazenil detox". This is supposed to wipe out your tolerance that has been built up and prevent withdrawal symptoms when the benzos are removed. There is debate on this one because of inconsistent results - i.e. - it works great for some and causes others to have suicidal ideation. Again, if you choose to try something like this, be sure to do your homework. Otherwise, tapering is highly recommended when you detox from Benzos.

If you've done some research online, you may have run across some groups that recommend "tapering" off your drug of choice before stopping completely. This is hotly debated when it comes to many different drugs but NOT with benzodiazepines. It is almost universally accepted by experts and those who have recovered from benzo addiction that tapering is the way to go. As with any other addictive substance, however, it is not always as easy to do as it is to lay out in black and white.

Say you are taking 20 benzos a week and someone recommends that you start tapering off and go to 18 a week. That may be easier said than done, especially if you have those other 2 in your possession. Regardless of your desire to "quit" or not, this is not an easy proposition and some are more successful with this than others. If you feel that you can trust someone else with your substances (many can't) and can have them rationed out to you, this may work. Otherwise, the craving may still get the best of you and you go straight to a source for more anyway. If you do decide to try tapering, here are some "**Hard Rules for Tapering**" that you will need to stick to:

1. Line up a tough trusted friend, spouse or significant other who will be in charge of your meds and will dole them out to you. This person will have to hold the line no matter how much you whine and try to manipulate.
2. Follow a set schedule. The schedule should be written out and turned over to the person administering the meds.
3. Approach the tapering from a clinical point of view (yes, I know this is difficult).
4. The heavier doses should be first thing in the morning and last of the evening
5. Do not attempt to delay a dosing time and hold off. This will cause a rebound effect that you don't want - i.e. - you will crave more.
6. Before starting your schedule, count up the exact number of pills you'll require from start to finish...and FLUSH all extraneous pills
7. Before starting your schedule, go to every hiding spot you have and discard those pills. Check jacket pockets, glove compartments, underwear drawers, shoes, handbags, etc. You get the idea. A nasty surprise after you've finished your taper is not something you want to encounter.
8. Hold nothing back "just in case". That's a reservation and it will do you in.
9. Do not rush the taper. Don't get brave. Brave is often foolish and looking for that instant gratification of instant "clean." It won't work.
10. No yo-yo-ing (spiking). An extra pill will interrupt your process and reset your progress. This is highly counter-productive. The goal is to titrate steadily downward.
11. No chewing or snorting. Take them the old fashioned way...with a glass of water and swallow.
12. Cut off all connections; that dealer, that doctor, that pharmacy...whomever, unless that doctor has become your

detox ally. They no longer exist for you. Shut the door firmly. Delete all numbers from your phone.

13. Have no expectation that this will be a comfortable process. Accept it for what it is...a rite of passage to freedom.

Because you are in one of these situations where tapering may be of benefit to you, consult your physician before starting. Even where other drugs are used in the detox process, they are tapered so as not to cause an additional dependence situation. Otherwise, keep in mind that addiction is a very powerful disease and tapering, by itself, is oftentimes easier said than done.

Benzo Detox Tapering Methods

Believe you can and you're halfway there. - Theodore Roosevelt

Tapering refers to slowly reducing the amount of the drug that you are taking over a period of time in order to lessen, or eliminate, withdrawal symptoms. With respect to Benzos, this is the recommended, and safest, course of action. The tough part comes in creating a specific plan for your detox and tapering based on your circumstances. An important thing to remember when putting your plan together for Benzo Detox is that it's better to reduce too slowly than to reduce too quickly. Several things to consider are: what drug(s) you are taking, quantity taken per day and length of time you have been taking the drugs. The third item is not as important as the first two but consider that someone that has been dependent upon Xanax for 3 months may have an easier time with detox than someone that has been taking it for 10 years.

Once it's established that you wish to taper from benzos, next you will need to decide which method you wish to use to do this. There are several choices: The Direct Taper, Substitution Taper (Ashton Method), and Titration.

Benzo Detox with a Direct Taper

A direct taper is often appropriate for the majority of people who have become addicted to benzos and involves tapering of the same medication - no substitutions. Therefore, if you have been taking Ativan for 10 years, you will taper off of that same drug until you "jump off" to nothing at all.

A direct taper approach generally involves making cuts of approximately 10% of the dose every one to two weeks. This is an estimate and it's important to understand that everyone's results will vary. Some people will have no trouble with this whatsoever and others will need to go at a slower pace, either with smaller cuts or more time between reductions. Putting a plan together before you start is crucial and also be prepared to make adjustments to the plan if needed.

As cuts are made, they are made as 10% of the current dose, not of the starting dose. Below is a 37 period (not week) schedule that can be used as an example for any benzo using a direct taper. You start with the number of tablets that you have for that 1 or 2 week period and then make the reductions per the table. For example, at period 37, you take 20 tablets with no reductions. After 1-2 weeks (you decide your schedule), you are down to 18 tablets for that period and you take 10% off of each of those, and so on.

Step No.	No. of tabs.	Percent cut		Step No.	No. of tabs.	Percent cut
BENZO FREE!						
1	1/4	50.00%		20	5 1/2	8.33%
2	1/2	33.33%		21	6	7.69%
3	3/4	25.00%		22	6 1/2	7.14%
4	1	20.00%		23	7	6.67%
5	1 1/4	16.67%		24	7 1/2	6.25%
6	1 1/2	14.29%		25	8	5.88%
7	1 3/4	12.50%		26	8 1/2	5.56%
8	2	11.11%		27	9	10.00%
9	2 1/4	10.00%		28	10	9.09%
10	2 1/2	9.09%		29	11	8.33%
11	2 3/4	8.33%		30	12	7.69%
12	3	7.69%		31	13	7.14%
13	3 1/4	7.14%		32	14	6.67%
14	3 1/2	6.67%		33	15	6.25%
15	3 3/4	6.25%		34	16	5.88%
16	4	5.88%		35	17	5.56%
17	4 1/4	5.56%		36	18	10.00%
18	4 1/2	10.00%		37	20	
19	5	9.09%				

There are a few things to keep in mind about this type of tapering. One is that it is the most straightforward but it doesn't work for everyone. When detoxing from short-acting benzos, it is sometimes better to use one of the other methods. Also, if you are going to use this method, switch to the lowest dose tablet available in your particular benzo. This makes cutting down much simpler. Finally, it's ok to hold off on moving to the next reduction in your schedule until you have recovered from the last one. However, it's never a good idea to increase or boost your dosage in an effort to recover from negative effects of withdrawal.

Benzo Detox with a Substitution Taper

A substitution taper involves substituting the patient's short-acting benzo, such as Lorazepam, for a long-acting benzo. This method is also often referred to as the "Ashton Method" in reference to Prof C Heather Ashton, who developed it. The first step is to figure out what you have been taking, total, on a daily basis. Once you have this information together, consider that you are going to be much more comfortable if you can "cross over" your current benzodiazepine use to the equivalent dose of Diazepam (aka - Valium). If your Benzo "of choice" is already Valium, no switching is needed. Here is the reason: **drug half life**. Many Benzos, like Xanax, are short acting and result in the rising and falling of the quantities of the medication in your bloodstream many times over the course of a day, which can lead to feelings of withdrawal and cravings. Longer acting medications, like Valium, result in more stable blood concentrations. Valium has a half life of up to 200 hours, meaning that the blood level for each dose falls by half in about 8.3 days. There are a few other similar Benzos but Valium (Diazepam) is also recommended because you can obtain it in 2mg tablets, which can also be halved to 1mg tabs if necessary.

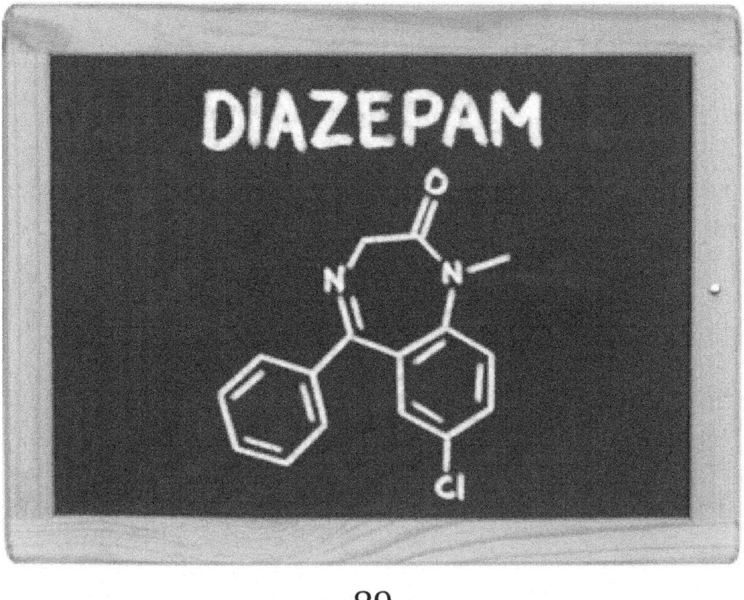

First let's take a look at the approximate equivalent dosages of Diazepam (Valium) for other Benzos that you may be taking:

The approximate equivalent dose to 10mg diazepam (Valium) are given below:

Benzodiazepines	Half-Life (hrs), [active metabolite]	Approximate Equivalent Oral Dosages (mg)
Alprazolam (Xanax)	6-12	0.5
Chlordiazepam (Librium)	5-30 [36-200]	5-6
Clonazepam (Klonopin, Rivotril)	18-50	0.5
Flunitrazepam (Rohypnol)	18-26 [36-200]	10
Lorazepam (Ativan)	10-20	1
Oxazepam (Serax, Serenid D)	4-15	20
Temazepam (Restoril)	8-22	20
Triazolam (Halcion)	2	0.5

For example, if you were taking 1mg of Ativan per day, this would be the equivalent of 10mg of Valium. 2mg of Halcion per day would be the equivalent of 40mg of Valium and 100mg of Restoril per day would be the equivalent of 50mg of Valium.

Now that we have that figured out, is it as simple as just switching out one for the other and then tapering off? No, not even close. Unfortunately, the "cross over" needs to be done in a gradual or step-wise fashion or there could be dire consequences. One reason for this is, though we gave you a fancy looking equivalency chart (above), these are not precise and the way that these metabolize in your body could be slightly different. Also, Valium may have a slightly different profile of action than the Benzo that you are used to taking, i.e. - perhaps less hypnotic activity. This may result in more or less sleepiness and a change in anxiety levels. This is why substitutions of Valium are done gradually over time and not all at once. Then, once you are exclusively on an equivalent dose of Valium, further tapering can begin. Again, the longer the better and the more time and thought that you put into your detox plan, the greater your chances for success and the better you'll be able to manage Benzo withdrawals, or avoid them altogether.

Here are some tapering examples used by actual patients that have detoxed from specific Benzos. These outline the schedule by which you would "cross over" gradually to the equivalent dose of Valium and the tapering schedule based on the Benzo being detoxed from. When viewing these schedules, remember that these are examples only and that every individual is different - has a different body chemistry, was likely on these drugs a different period of time than you were and may have, or not have, other physical and/or mental conditions that affected the outcome of this. In other words, this is absolutely not medical advice and you would be wise to consult your physician before moving forward. Benzo Tapering Examples:

Table 1 - Withdrawal from Lorazepam (Ativan) 6mg/day:

Withdrawal from lorazepam (Ativan) 6mg daily with diazepam (Valium) substitution. (6mg lorazepam is approximately equivalent to 60mg diazepam)				
	Morning	**Midday/ Afternoon**	**Evening /Night**	**Daily Diazepam Equivalent**
Starting dosage	lorazepam 2mg	lorazepam 2mg	lorazepam 2mg	60mg
Stage 1 (one week)	lorazepam 2mg	lorazepam 2mg	lorazepam 1mg diazepam 10mg	60mg
Stage 2 (one week)	lorazepam 1.5mg diazepam 5mg	lorazepam 2mg	lorazepam 1mg diazepam 10mg	60mg
Stage 3 (one week)	lorazepam 1.5mg diazepam 5mg	lorazepam 2mg	lorazepam 0.5mg diazepam 15mg	60mg
Stage 4 (one week)	lorazepam 1.5mg diazepam 5mg	lorazepam 1.5mg diazepam 5mg	lorazepam 0.5mg diazepam 15mg	60mg
Stage 5 (1-2 weeks)	lorazepam 1.5mg diazepam 5mg	lorazepam 1.5mg diazepam 5mg	Stop lorazepam diazepam 20mg	60mg
Stage 6 (1-2 weeks)	lorazepam 1mg diazepam 5mg	lorazepam 1.5mg diazepam 5mg	diazepam 20mg	55mg
Stage 7 (1-2 weeks)	lorazepam 1mg diazepam 5mg	lorazepam 1mg diazepam 5mg	diazepam 20mg	50mg
Stage 8 (1-2 weeks)	lorazepam 0.5mg diazepam 5mg	lorazepam 1mg diazepam 5mg	diazepam 20mg	45mg
Stage 9 (1-2 weeks)	lorazepam 0.5mg diazepam 5mg	lorazepam 0.5mg diazepam 5mg	diazepam 20mg	40mg
Stage 10 (1-2 weeks)	Stop lorazepam diazepam 5mg	lorazepam 0.5mg diazepam 5mg	diazepam 20mg	35mg
Stage 11 (1-2 weeks)	diazepam 5mg	Stop lorazepam diazepam 5mg	diazepam 20mg	30mg
Stage 12 (1-2 weeks)	diazepam 5mg	diazepam 5mg	diazepam 18mg	28mg
Stage 13 (1-2 weeks)	diazepam 5mg	diazepam 5mg	diazepam 16mg	26mg
Stage 14 (1-2 weeks)	diazepam 5mg	diazepam 5mg	diazepam 14mg	24mg
Stage 15 (1-2 weeks)	diazepam 5mg	diazepam 5mg	diazepam 12mg	22mg
Stage 16 (1-2 weeks)	diazepam 5mg	diazepam 5mg	diazepam 10mg	20mg

	Morning	Midday/ Afternoon	Evening /Night	Daily Diazepam Equivalent
Stage 17 (1-2 weeks)	diazepam 5mg	diazepam 4mg	diazepam 10mg	19mg
Stage 18 (1-2 weeks)	diazepam 4mg	diazepam 4mg	diazepam 10mg	18mg
Stage 19 (1-2 weeks)	diazepam 4mg	diazepam 3mg	diazepam 10mg	17mg
Stage 20 (1-2 weeks)	diazepam 3mg	diazepam 3mg	diazepam 10mg	16mg
Stage 21 (1-2 weeks)	diazepam 3mg	diazepam 2mg	diazepam 10mg	15mg
Stage 22 (1-2 weeks)	diazepam 2mg	diazepam 2mg	diazepam 10mg	14mg
Stage 23 (1-2 weeks)	diazepam 2mg	diazepam 1mg	diazepam 10mg	13mg
Stage 24 (1-2 weeks)	diazepam 1mg	diazepam 1mg	diazepam 10mg	12mg
Stage 25 (1-2 weeks)	diazepam 1mg	Stop diazepam	diazepam 10mg	11mg
Stage 26 (1-2 weeks)	Stop diazepam	--	diazepam 10mg	10mg
Stage 27 (1-2 weeks)	--	--	diazepam 9mg	9mg
Stage 28 (1-2 weeks)	--	--	diazepam 8mg	8mg
Stage 29 (1-2 weeks)	--	--	diazepam 7mg	7mg
Stage 30 (1-2 weeks)	--	--	diazepam 6mg	6mg
Stage 31 (1-2 weeks)	--	--	diazepam 5mg	5mg
Stage 32 (1-2 weeks)	--	--	diazepam 4mg	4mg
Stage 33 (1-2 weeks)	--	--	diazepam 3mg	3mg
Stage 34 (1-2 weeks)	--	--	diazepam 2mg	2mg
Stage 35 (1-2 weeks)	--	--	diazepam 1mg	1mg
Stage 36	--	--	Stop diazepam	--

Table 2: Withdrawal from Alprazolam (Xanax) 6mg/day:

Withdrawal from high dose (6mg) alprazolam (Xanax daily with diazepam (Valium) substitution. (6mg alprazolam is approximately equivalent to 120mg diazepam)				
	Morning	**Midday/ Afternoon**	**Evening /Night**	**Daily Diazepam Equivalent**
Starting dosage	alprazolam 2mg	alprazolam 2mg	alprazolam 2mg	120mg
Stage 1 (one week)	alprazolam 2mg	alprazolam 2mg	alprazolam 1.5mg diazepam 10mg	120mg
Stage 2 (one week)	alprazolam 2mg	alprazolam 2mg	alprazolam 1mg diazepam 20mg	120mg
Stage 3 (one week)	alprazolam 1.5mg diazepam 10mg	alprazolam 2mg	alprazolam 1mg diazepam 20mg	120mg
Stage 4 (one week)	alprazolam 1mg diazepam 20mg	alprazolam 2mg	alprazolam 1mg diazepam 20mg	120mg
Stage 5 (1-2 weeks)	alprazolam 1mg diazepam 20mg	alprazolam 1mg diazepam 10mg	alprazolam 1mg diazepam 20mg	110mg
Stage 6 (1-2 weeks)	alprazolam 1mg diazepam 20mg	alprazolam 1mg diazepam 10mg	alprazolam 0.5mg diazepam 20mg	100mg
Stage 7 (1-2 weeks)	alprazolam 1mg diazepam 20mg	alprazolam 1mg diazepam 10mg	Stop alprazolam diazepam 20mg	90mg
Stage 8 (1-2 weeks)	alprazolam 0.5mg diazepam 20mg	alprazolam 1mg diazepam 10mg	diazepam 20mg	80mg
Stage 9 (1-2 weeks)	alprazolam 0.5mg diazepam 20mg	alprazolam 0.5mg diazepam 10mg	diazepam 20mg	80mg
Stage 10 (1-2 weeks)	alprazolam 0.5mg diazepam 20mg	Stop alprazolam diazepam 10mg	diazepam 20mg	60mg
Stage 11 (1-2 weeks)	Stop alprazolam diazepam 20mg	diazepam 10mg	diazepam 20mg	50mg
Stage 12 (1-2 weeks)	diazepam 25mg	Stop midday dose;	diazepam 25mg	50mg

	Morning	Midday/ Afternoon	Evening /Night	Daily Diazepam Equivalent
Stage 13 (1-2 weeks)	diazepam 20mg	--	diazepam 25mg	45mg
Stage 14 (1-2 weeks)	diazepam 20mg	--	diazepam 20mg	40mg
Stage 15 (1-2 weeks)	diazepam 20mg	--	diazepam 20mg	40mg
Stage 16 (1-2 weeks)	diazepam 18mg	--	diazepam 20mg	38mg
Stage 17 (1-2 weeks)	diazepam 18mg	--	diazepam 18mg	36mg
Stage 18 (1-2 weeks)	diazepam 16mg	--	diazepam 18mg	34mg
Stage 19 (1-2 weeks)	diazepam 16mg	--	diazepam 16mg	32mg
Stage 20 (1-2 weeks)	diazepam 14mg	--	diazepam 16mg	30mg
Stage 21 (1-2 weeks)	diazepam 14mg	--	diazepam 14mg	28mg
Stage 22 (1-2 weeks)	diazepam 12mg	--	diazepam 14mg	26mg
Stage 23 (1-2 weeks)	diazepam 12mg	--	diazepam 12mg	24mg
Stage 24 (1-2 weeks)	diazepam 10mg	--	diazepam 12mg	22mg
Stage 25 (1-2 weeks)	diazepam 10mg	--	diazepam 10mg	20mg
Stage 26 (1-2 weeks)	diazepam 8mg	--	diazepam 10mg	18mg
Stage 27 (1-2 weeks)	diazepam 8mg	--	diazepam 8mg	16mg

	Morning	Midday/ Afternoon	Evening /Night	Daily Diazepam Equivalent
Stage 28 (1-2 weeks)	diazepam 6mg	--	diazepam 8mg	14mg
Stage 29 (1-2 weeks)	diazepam 5mg	--	diazepam 8mg	13mg
Stage 30 (1-2 weeks)	diazepam 4mg	--	diazepam 8mg	12mg
Stage 31 (1-2 weeks)	diazepam 3mg	--	diazepam 8mg	11mg
Stage 32 (1-2 weeks)	diazepam 2mg	--	diazepam 8mg	10mg
Stage 33 (1-2 weeks)	diazepam 1mg	--	diazepam 8mg	9mg
Stage 34 (1-2 weeks)	--	--	diazepam 8mg	8mg
Stage 35 (1-2 weeks)	--	--	diazepam 7mg	7mg
Stage 36 (1-2 weeks)	--	--	diazepam 6mg	6mg
Stage 37 (1-2 weeks)	--	--	diazepam 5mg	5mg
Stage 38 (1-2 weeks)	--	--	diazepam 4mg	4mg
Stage 39 (1-2 weeks)	--	--	diazepam 3mg	3mg
Stage 40 (1-2 weeks)	--	--	diazepam 2mg	2mg
Stage 41 (1-2 weeks)	--	--	diazepam 1mg	1mg
	--	--	Stop diazepam	--

Table 3: Withdrawal from Clonazepam (Klonopin) 1.5mg/day:

Withdrawal from clonazepam (Klonopin) 1.5mg daily with substitution of diazepam (Valium). (0.5mg clonazepam is approximately equivalent to 10mg diazepam)				
	Morning	**Midday/ Afternoon**	**Evening /Night**	**Daily Diazepam Equivalent**
Starting dosage	clonazepam 0.5mg	clonazepam 0.5mg	clonazepam 0.5mg	30mg
Stage 1 (1 week)	clonazepam 0.5mg	clonazepam 0.5mg	0.25mg diazepam 5mg	30mg
Stage 2 (1 week)	clonazepam 0.5mg	clonazepam 0.5mg	Stop clonazepam diazepam 10mg	30mg
Stage 3 (1 week)	clonazepam 0.25mg diazepam 5mg	clonazepam 0.5mg	diazepam 10mg	30mg
Stage 4 (1 week)	clonazepam 0.25mg diazepam 5mg	clonazepam 0.25mg diazepam 5mg	diazepam 10mg	30mg
Stage 5 (1 week)	Stop clonazepam diazepam 10mg	clonazepam 0.25mg diazepam 5mg	diazepam 10mg	30mg
Stage 6 (1-2 weeks)	diazepam 10mg	Stop clonazepam diazepam 8mg	diazepam 10mg	28mg
Stage 7 (1-2 weeks)	diazepam 10mg	diazepam 6mg	diazepam 10mg	26mg
Stage 8 (1-2 weeks)	diazepam 10mg	diazepam 4mg	diazepam 10mg	24mg
Stage 9 (1-2 weeks)	diazepam 10mg	diazepam 2mg	diazepam 10mg	22mg
Stage 10 (1-2 weeks)	diazepam 10mg	Stop diazepam	diazepam 10mg	20mg
Stage 11 (1-2 weeks)	diazepam 8mg	--	diazepam 10mg	18mg

	Morning	Midday/ Afternoon	Evening /Night	Daily Diazepam Equivalent
Stage 12 (1-2 weeks)	diazepam 6mg	--	diazepam 10mg	16mg
Stage 13 (1-2 weeks)	diazepam 4mg	--	diazepam 10mg	14mg
Stage 14 (1-2 weeks)	diazepam 2mg	--	diazepam 10mg	12mg
Stage 15 (1-2 weeks)	Stop diazepam	--	diazepam 10mg	10mg
Stage 16 (1-2 weeks)	--	--	diazepam 9mg	9mg
Stage 17 (1-2 weeks)	--	--	diazepam 8mg	8mg
Stage 18 (1-2 weeks)	--	--	diazepam 7mg	7mg
Stage 19 (1-2 weeks)	--	--	diazepam 6mg	6mg
Stage 20 (1-2 weeks)	--	--	diazepam 5mg	5mg
Stage 21 (1-2 weeks)	--	--	diazepam 4mg	4mg
Stage 22 (1-2 weeks)	--	--	diazepam 3mg	3mg
Stage 23 (1-2 weeks)	--	--	diazepam 2mg	2mg
Stage 24 (1-2 weeks)	--	--	diazepam 1mg	1mg
	--	--	Stop diazepam	--

Table 4: Withdrawal from Temazepam (Restoril) 30mg/day (taken at night):

Withdrawal from temazepam (Restoril) 30mg nightly with diazepam substitution. (30mg temazepam is approximately equivalent to 15mg diazepam)		
	Evening /Night	Daily Diazepam Equivalent
Starting dosage	temazepam 30mg	15mg
Stage 1 (1-2 weeks)	temazepam 15mg diazepam 7.5mg	15mg
Stage 2 (1-2 weeks)	temazepam 7.5mg diazepam 12mg	15.75mg
Stage 3 (1-2 weeks)	Stop temazepam diazepam 15mg	15mg
Stage 4 (1-2 weeks)	diazepam 14mg	14mg
Stage 5 (1-2 weeks)	diazepam 13mg	13mg
Stage 6 (1-2 weeks)	diazepam 12mg	12mg
Stage 7 (1-2 weeks)	diazepam 11mg	11mg
Stage 8 (1-2 weeks)	diazepam 10mg	10mg
Stage 9 (1-2 weeks)	diazepam 9mg	9mg
Stage 10 (1-2 weeks)	diazepam 8mg	8mg
Stage 11 (1-2 weeks)	diazepam 7mg	7mg
Stage 12 (1-2 weeks)	diazepam 6mg	6mg
Stage 13 (1-2 weeks)	diazepam 5mg	5mg
Stage 14 (1-2 weeks)	diazepam 4mg	4mg
Stage 15 (1-2 weeks)	diazepam 3mg	3mg
Stage 16 (1-2 weeks)	diazepam 2mg	2mg
Stage 17 (1-2 weeks)	diazepam 1mg	1mg
Stage 18	Stop diazepam	--

A few things about substitution tapering that are notable. One is that this can be implemented at any time during your taper, meaning that you could be doing a straight taper, decide that it's not working for you and make the decision to switch to this one. The other is that it's ok, as with the other method, to take it slow and make adjustments as needed during the process. This isn't an exact science and everyone's body and brain react differently. If you have difficulty with the daily schedule, even if you only took benzos once a day when they were prescribed, it's ok to adjust this during the detox process as long as you are not increasing the overall daily dose.

Benzo Detox with a Triration Taper

In medical circles, the term triration refers to an analysis technique in which one solution of a known concentration is slowly added to an unknown concentration until the reaction reaches neutralization. While a great science lesson for us, that's not what we're referring to at all when we talk about a triration detox. In detox, water or milk is added to benzo tablets to create a liquid benzodiazepine, which is then utilized to make small, intricate cuts to dosages.

While this many sound daunting, this method is actually quite useful in several cases. One is for anyone who simply cannot understand or follow the other tapering schedules because of the math involved. This is one of the more straightforward methods because there is a website (benzobuddies.org) that will actually do all of the work for you and provided you with a personalized schedule to follow. The instance that this method may be useful is when you are taking very small doses of benzos and the reductions, or pill-splitting, become very difficult. That being said, there is still work to do with this one as you are crushing pills in a mortar and making liquid benzodiazepine on a daily basis. If that doesn't appeal to you, you may want to skip this method.

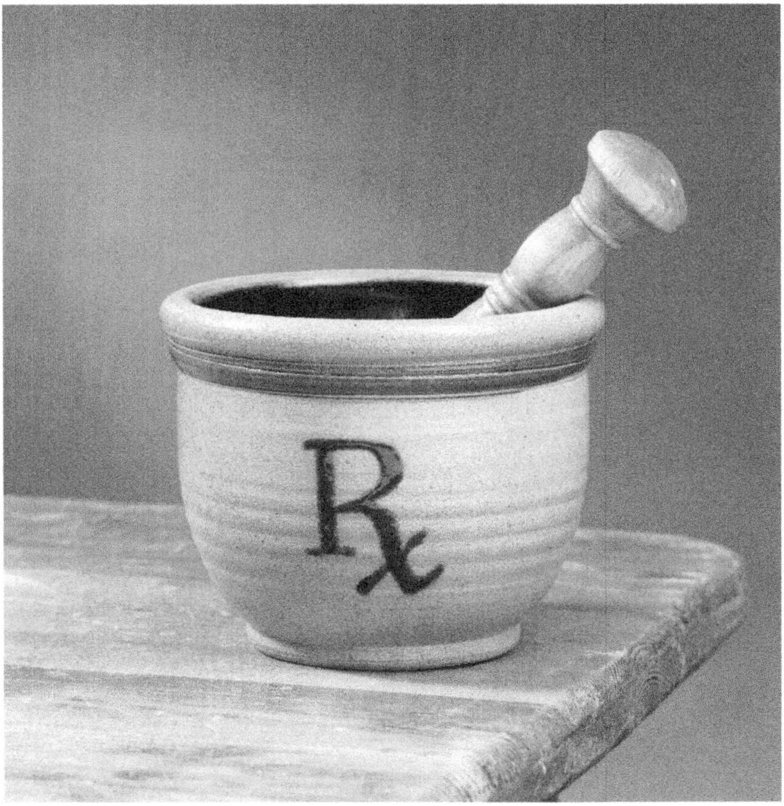
Rx

What to Expect When You Detox From Benzodiazepines

If anything has gotten through to you so far, hopefully it is that this is not something to take lightly or jump into without a lot of thought and planning. Even with the "cross over" and tapering, expect that you will experience at least some discomfort and withdrawal symptoms. The onset of withdrawal from benzos depends on the half-life of the particular drug that you were taking. Once that half-life has elapsed and you haven't taken another pill, symptoms will appear and shorter acting benzodiazepines tend to have more severe withdrawal symptoms. Duration of acute phase of symptoms can range from 4-8 weeks, or longer, and may include:

- Anxiety
- Tinnitus
- Tremors
- Insomnia
- Perceptual distortion
- Muscle cramps, muscle twitching
- Paranoia
- Paraesthesia
- Convulsions
- Headache
- Confusion, disorientation
- Nausea, vomiting
- Hallucinations
- Fatigue

Benzos were often prescribed in the first place for anxiety and these feelings have a tendency to return quite quickly once the drugs are removed. This is also why tapering is important. Craving for the drugs can persist for weeks or even months. Benzodiazepines also offer a set of symptoms that are unique to this class of drugs, called

Post-Acute Withdrawal Symptoms (PAWS) that we talk about later in this section. If you reviewed those sample schedules, you can see that a long tapering schedule can last anywhere from 6-18 months. Be patient with yourself and you'll be much better off in the long run.

While the road ahead may seem tough, if you have gone through the exercise at the beginning of the book where you take a look at why you are doing this and what you stand to gain, you'll be able to see the light at the end of the tunnel already. There are still other preparations that you can make beforehand to make your detox much more comfortable.

Preparation for Benzodiazepine Detox at Home

Find a place inside where there's joy, and the joy will burn out the pain. -Joseph Campbell

If you are planning to detox from Benzos at home, be sure to review the general home detox guide earlier in this section about putting together a detox plan and setting up some support. Aside from that, you'll need to make some special preparations with respect to detoxing from Benzos at home.

Prepare the Environment

It would be at this point that I would generally tell you to take some time off of work, send the kids away and rent a bunch of movies to pass the time that you will be "holed up" in your home. Not so in this case. In fact, if you are going to need to take some time off and "lay low", it may not be until the very end of the process where you are actually removing the long-acting Valium from your body and may feel crummy and very tired for several days. In general, if you are sticking to a nice slow, long tapering schedule, you should be able to continue with your daily schedule of activities, including work. Don't expect life to be "fun" for awhile, but it should be manageable and safe. That's the point of doing this slowly.

Support

Involving your physician in this endeavor is critical. As soon as you commit to detoxing from Benzos and doing this "at home", you need to schedule an appointment with your doctor and let him/her know your plan and request what you need from them. Specifically, you'll want to discuss any other medical or psychological conditions that may interfere with a home detox and also discuss a tapering schedule using Diazepam (Valium) if you are going to do a Substitution Taper. Set a date to start the process and schedule a follow up appointment with your physician sometime in the first 1-2 weeks to discuss progress.

It would also be a good idea to enlist other people to act as "support" pillars in your detox project. Whether it be family members or close friends, let someone else know what you are doing and why you are doing it. If you think no one knows what has been going on with you, you'd be surprised to find out that the secret has been out for quite some time and that the people that love you really only want the best for you in the end. They'll be supportive and willing to help in any way. You may need help in "doling" out medications so that you aren't tempted to take more than is on your tapering schedule or maybe you just need some encouragement. Either way, get started in setting that up now.

There really are no over the counter meds or other prescriptions that are recommended to help with Benzo detox. There are occasionally prescriptions given to address certain symptoms if they are severe enough and these would need to be managed by your physician. These include Anti-Depressants and Beta Blockers. Otherwise, it's highly cautioned that you not turn to other substances, like alcohol or marijuana, in an effort to ease symptoms as this will just cause more problems later on. However, you will want to increase your vitamin and mineral intake and you can start by picking up some of the following:

- Vitamin C
- Vitamin D

- Magnesium
- L-Glutamine
- Melatonin
- Milk Thistle
- Omega3 (ex - Fish Oil)

Diet

When we are anticipating not feeling well, we may be inclined to grab a bunch of "comfort foods" as they are sure to make us feel better and get us through a rough time. In this case, that would be a mistake. Cookies and candy are not going to give our heart and liver the nutrients that they need as they is over-working to detoxify our body from these mass amounts of toxins that have built up in it. You'll want to reduce the load on your liver by minimizing the processed foods and saturated fats that you put in your body. While detoxing from benzos, generally your appetite will go back and forth. Some days you may not have an appetite at all and others you may be very hungry. If you're not feeling well, it's ok to eat in small amounts but when you do eat something, eat the right things. Either way, stock up on some of this stuff:

- Fiber-rich fruits and vegetables
- Healthy proteins from chicken, fish and eggs
- Plant proteins such as beans and peas
- Healthy fats from fish
- Nuts, seeds, extra virgin olive oil

An interesting thing about many psyche drugs, benzos included, is that they tend to lower histamine in the body and make the user sensitive to foods that they may not have had an issue with in the past. Those who do have histamine issues cannot eat bone broths or many cultured foods as they aren't appealing, lower energy levels and can have a tendency to affect withdrawal symptoms. While not entirely proven to date, this is something to take a closer look at.

Also, fluid intake is very important during detox and withdrawal. Drink a ton of water every day. Stay away from excess amounts of soda and coffee for at least a few weeks if you can. This isn't as crucial as with some of the other detoxes as you may be overly tired at times. So, if you would like an occasional cup of coffee, that's probably ok but keep it to that. Green tea is also ok to drink and is good for its antioxidants and anti inflammatory properties. It's ok to have a few sports drinks for flavor but stick mostly to good old fashioned water - and lots of it.

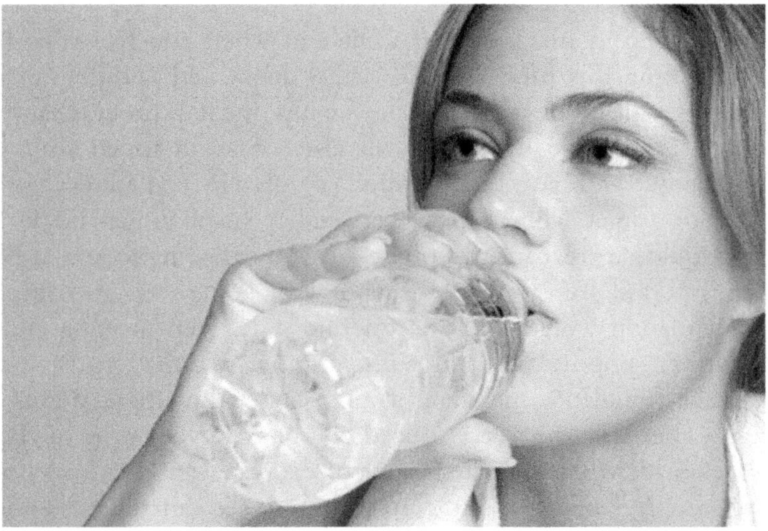

Other Activities

It's ok to sleep as much as you want and when you feel your body needs it during this process. However, detox and withdrawal from benzos is both a physical and a highly mental process and it's important to manage this above all else. Stay in touch with your support people and have them remind of you why you are doing this - we tend to forget when times get tough. Inspirational books and movies would be great for this process if you are going to stay at home for any period of time. If you are going to go out, the recommendation would be that you find a 12 Step meeting and get some further support there. Again, it's imperative that you stay away from other stimulants, including alcohol and other drugs, during this process. They will only serve to lead you back to your drug of choice. Finally, consider that a small amount of exercise can go a long way in making you feel better. Just a 10 minute walk can release some of those endorphins that are no longer being released by the drugs and give you a sense of well-being. Do this each day and you will be amazed at the results.

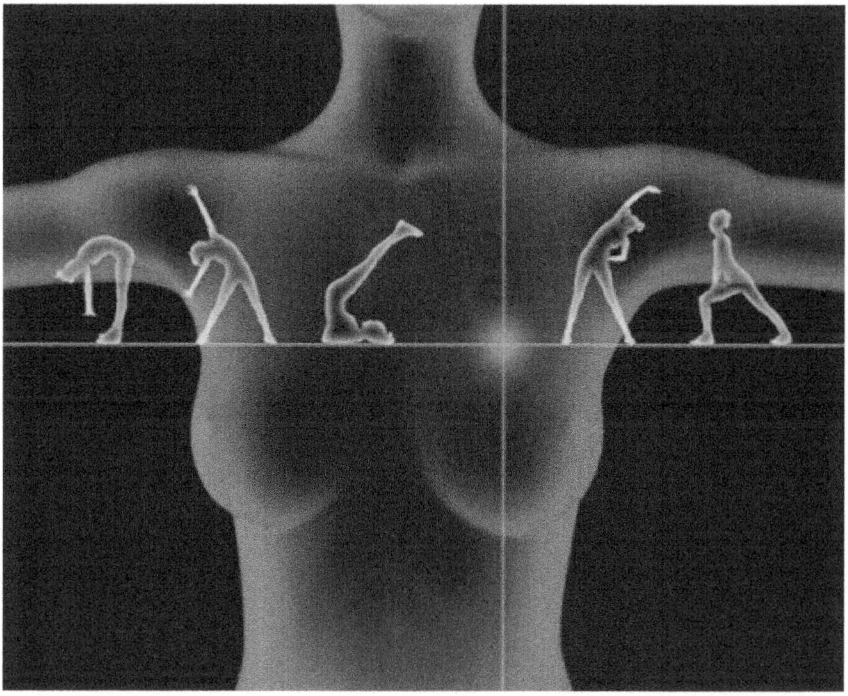

Post Acute Withdrawal Symptoms

It was not long before I discovered that withdrawing addicts lost their composure in exactly the same manner that careless millionaires lose their money: gradually, then suddenly. — Andrew Davidson

Post Acute Withdrawal Syndrome (PAWS), also known as protracted withdrawal syndrome, is a delayed set of symptoms that hit about 10%-15% of benzo addicts, after the acute phase of detox has passed. These symptoms can appear anytime after withdrawal has completed and last for months or even years. The syndrome represents a combination of both psychological and pharmacological factors directly related to benzodiazepine use.

One of the unique things about PAWS and benzos is the potential for duration and severity of symptoms. PAWS are actually defined as symptoms that are significant, debilitating, and continuous. So, if your symptoms are occasional and mild, it's likely not PAWS. It can also become difficult at times to distinguish between PAWS and the recurrence of an underlying condition. Some common PAWS symptoms include:

- Anxiety
- Insomnia
- Depression
- Perceptual symptoms: tinnitus, paraesthesiae — tingling, numbness, pain usually in limbs, extremities
- Motor symptoms: muscle pain, weakness, tension, painful cramps, tremor, shaking attacks, jerks, blepharospasm

- Gastro-intestinal symptoms
- Mechanisms for protracted symptoms not known, but may include both psychological and pharmacological factors, and possibly structural brain damage.

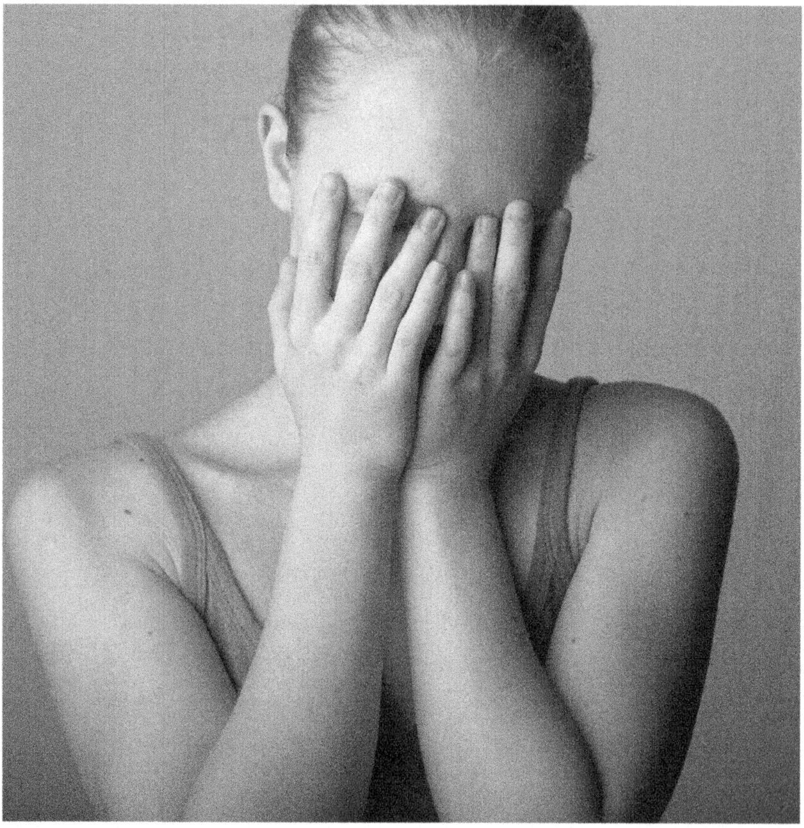

Roger's Story:

I endured 18 months of benzo withdrawal – whereby every day I awoke feeling like I had the flu: aches, malaise, lethargy, and a debilitating foggy head. I exercised, read, attended support groups, and surrounded myself with family. It was very, very difficult.

The acute phase of benzo withdrawal syndrome is generally classified to last anywhere from 5 to 28 days and PAWS is something that can kick in at any time after that, lasting months, and even years for some symptoms. While a terrifying prospect on the surface, there are a few important points to get across about PAWS with regards to benzos. First, even if you are in the category of people with a serious dependency, the statistical likelihood of you experiencing PAWS is quite small, probably less than 1 in 10. If you are two years out and have occasional, mild symptoms, that is not PAWS. It is typical. If you have significant, debilitating symptoms beyond a year, that is PAWS and it is atypical but not unheard of. However, the second thing to keep in mind is that there is no evidence that benzodiazepine withdrawal syndrome can ever be permanent. Even in the rare cases that symptoms persist for years, they gradually diminish over time until they are gone.

As you taper, do not concern yourself with whether or not you will experience PAWS. You probably will not. And even if you do, that is something to manage if or when you get there. Hopefully, this eases your mind a bit. One thing you should be prepared for, even though it is not an issue for many with benzos, are potential cravings for the drug and its effects.

Some Tips on Dealing With Cravings

Do not confuse your cravings with your needs - Renji George

Cravings are urges to drink or use drugs (yes, even legal ones). These urges are a normal part of any addiction and are common-place during withdrawal. They can also pop up months or even years after you stop using drugs or drinking. Others get free of benzos and never have another craving for them again, simply keeping in mind the hell that they were put through as a result of them. That's all well and good but preparation for what could show up on your doorstep is always the best defense. Here are some important things to remember about cravings and some ways to deal with them.

What You Should Know About Cravings:

- They are not caused by a lack of willpower or motivation. It doesn't mean that you are doing something wrong or failing to do something right.
- Cravings don't mean that your detox and withdrawal aren't working.
- Cravings pass. These urges are not constant and are only severe for a very short period of time before they settle down to a more controllable level.
- Cravings can be triggered by physical or psychological discomfort. Managing these can help manage the onset and severity of cravings.

Things You Can Do to Manage Cravings:

- Remind yourself that cravings are "temporary". In fact, if the urge to use is very strong, simply put the decision off for an hour and the feelings will likely subside.
- Identify cues or "triggers" that may have brought on the cravings. They could people, places or things that remind you of using. Re-direct your mental energy towards ways in which you can avoid these same triggers in the future.
- Remind yourself of why you stopped taking the drug in the first place. This would be the time to re-list the negative effects that the drug and/or alcohol use had on your life and also list the positive things that you stand to gain by staying clean.
- Call on others for help. This is where a Support Network comes in, supportive family members and friends that support your recovery.
- Use your spirituality to get through cravings. Prayer and meditation can help calm the mind and bring focus back into what you have achieved so far and what lies ahead in your recovery.

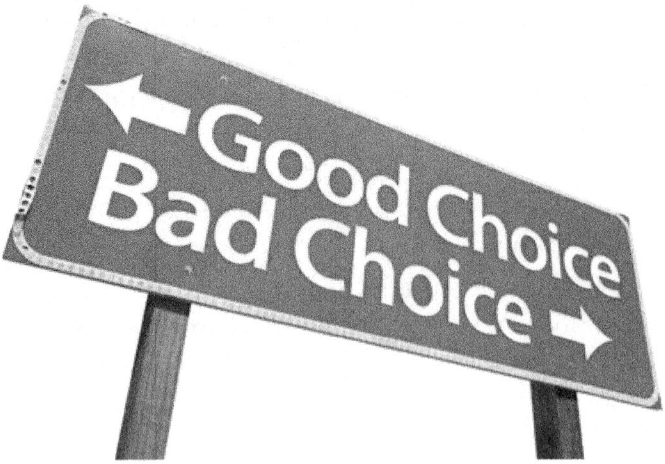

After Benzo Detox

Try to be like the turtle - at ease in your own shell. -Bill Copeland

---

The acute phase of Benzodiazepine withdrawal can be over in as little as 30 days after the last pill. That's just it though, the withdrawal phase and the residual toxins leaving your body. Compared to some of the other detox processes, this was a very long one and it would be a shame to screw it up and go back to the endless cycle of Benzodiazepine addiction. The detox certainly wasn't fun but all of that suffering would be for nothing if you were to walk right back out into the "real world" and resume using. Cravings can continue to be intense and a benzo habit is incredibly hard to break, almost impossible to do alone. This is why digesting the following information is so important:

Addiction is a bona fide disease (Read the Disease Chapter coming up - this is important)
Additional help or treatment is available and probably recommended (there is a Chapter on this as well)
Finding a good support network is critical to remaining clean long term (Also in this Section).

Otherwise, you have successfully detoxed from benzos at home. Maybe this wasn't the first time. Regardless, it more than likely wasn't fun and not something that you would want to repeat or even do over and over again. If that's the case, please check out those final chapters in the book and the Resource Section before moving on. Now that we've covered some basic things to know about detoxing from benzos, tapering and managing cravings, let's get into what you need to know about long-term recovery from benzodiazepine addiction.

Kerrie's Story:

Compared to many benzo addicts, my 5-month ordeal is nothing. What we endure during a few weeks of tapering or dealing with PAWS is more than many people deal with in a lifetime. One thing is for sure though, once we do triumph, there isn't much we can't handle. Our hurts and pains make us who we are and, in turn, make us stronger. I've seen some changes within myself that make me a better and stronger person. You will too. I've often thought that I would like to forget the rough times, but it's those times where my family stepped-up and that's not something I never want to forget. My journey was bitter-sweet in that aspect... Just know that your day will come and you will be standing on top of the world when it does.

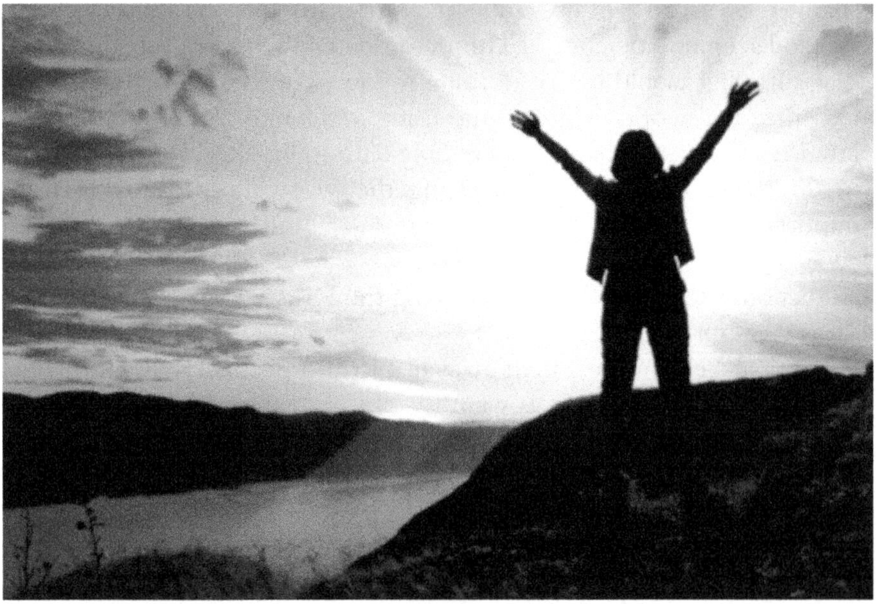

Life After Detox - Stop the Madness Merry-Go-Round

If we don't change our direction, we are likely to end up where we are headed. -Ancient Chinese Proverb

---

If this is your first go around with a Detox experience, be glad that it's over. Don't stop reading though as there are some important things that you need to consider, some "hard facts" if you will. If you've been through this before, the following will likely not come as much of a surprise to you, yet the reminders may do you some good and, hopefully, send you in the right direction this time. The fact of the matter is that simply getting the drugs out of our system isn't enough to recover from addiction. Many of us, myself included, have suffered from the delusions that we were simply trapped in a "physical addiction" and, once free, would be able to resume living life just as we had before all of this nonsense started. Wrong! There is an "invisible line" that has been crossed and you will never be able to go back to that "old life". That's the bad news. The good news is that you absolutely can recover from this and lead an even better life than you had ever imagined. Yes, it sounds ridiculous and like a bunch of "hocus pocus" right now, but stick with me here. There is light at the end of the tunnel after a bit more education and self discovery.

The mentality and behavior of drug addicts and alcoholics is wholly irrational until you understand that they are completely powerless over their addiction and unless they have structured help, they have no hope. — Russell Brand

---

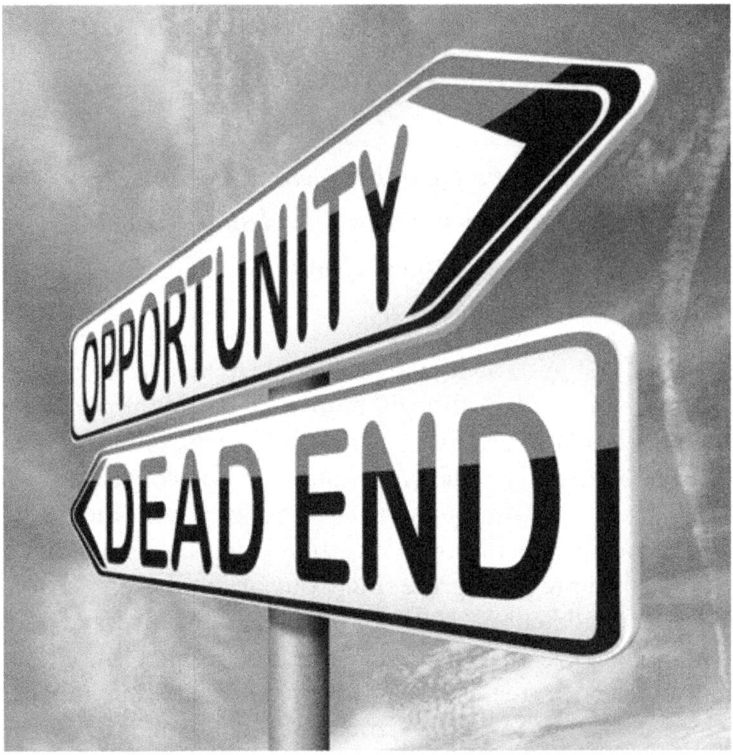
OPPORTUNITY
DEAD END

Understanding that Addiction is a Disease

It ain't what you don't know that gets you into trouble. It's what you know for sure that just ain't so. -Mark Twain

A fact that most addicts and alcoholics are in the dark about is that they actually have a "disease" and are not simply bad people that can't control themselves. In fact, for over 100 years, alcoholism has been treated as and defined as a "disease". In 1956, the American Medical Association voted to define alcoholism as a disease and, according to the National Institute on Drug Abuse (NIDA), "Addiction is defined as a chronic, relapsing brain disease that is characterized by compulsive drug seeking and use, despite harmful consequences." The American Society of Addiction Medicine (ASAM) also recently revised its definition of addiction to state that: "Addiction is a chronic brain disorder, and not merely a behavioral problem or simply the result of taking the wrong choices". Addiction is now described as a primary disease - not caused by something else, such as a psychiatric or emotional problem. Dr. Michael Miller, former president of ASAM, who oversaw the development of the new definition, said: "At its core, addiction isn't just a social problem or a moral problem or a criminal problem. It's a brain problem whose behaviors manifest in all these other areas. Many behaviors driven by addiction are real problems and sometimes criminal acts. But the disease is about brains, not drugs. It's about underlying neurology, not outward actions."

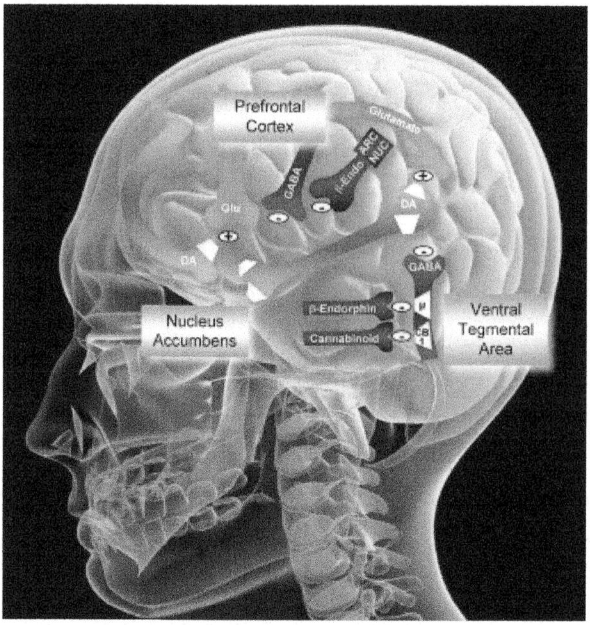

Again, many who read this book are going to want to know about how this relates to the situation of the "accidental addict". Sometimes referred in medical circles as iatrogenic addiction, this is an addiction that is "induced inadvertently by a physician or surgeon or by medical treatment or diagnostic procedures." The cause of the addiction may be much different than the heroin addicts or the alcoholic's but, for many, the end result is the same. In fact, the motivation for starting a psychotropic drug in the first place is often quite similar to that of the habitual drug user - the desire to change the way you feel.

The fact that the addiction itself was an "accident", can often give the addict justification for feelings and behaviors that aren't serving their best interests. No one likes the stigma of addiction and, if told that there may be an "out", any addict is going to grasp for that with their last dying breath. I know I did and it nearly killed me. In my opinion, the term "accidental addict" is a disservice to those who are going through this as it often prevents them from seeking treatment and getting the help that could save their lives. I've said it before that there are a small percentage of benzo addicts who can just stop taking these after detox and never think about them again. Why would you want to make such a high stakes gamble?

A few additional characteristics of the disease of Addiction (and Alcoholism - same thing) to be aware of are:

Mental Obsession - Defined as a thought process over which you have no control. Sounds like fun, right? These maddening urges to use or drink, when many times we know that the results will be disastrous. I always call this the "preoccupation" that I always had with when I would be able to get that next drink or drug - or how I would be able to get more than my "share".
Chronic Disease - By chronic, we mean that it is "incurable" (keep reading anyway) and requires long-term treatment. This is a disease that can also result in death if not treated.
Progressive - This one is important. (Well, the other two were also.) Addiction and Alcoholism is a subtly progressive disease that gets worse over time - NEVER better. Sometimes, this takes place over such an extended period of time that the addict does not notice the point at which they truly lost control. And, you know what? It doesn't matter. Because as soon as that control is "lost", it can NEVER be regained. EVER. This is where the difficulty and the denial come into play for so many. We remember that time when things were great, fun, easy, controllable and try with all our might, sometimes for entirely too long, to recapture it. It just won't happen.

So what does all of this new-found knowledge mean for the "addicted" or stricken person? Well, the good news is that you're "sick"! Yes, in this case, consider this good news. Think of it in these terms: you no longer need look at yourself as a bad person or an evil person who has screwed up their life and can't control themselves. The truth is that you are a "sick person" who simply needs to take some steps to get well. This is entirely possible and well within your reach if it is something that you want. While there is no cure per se for addiction, this is a disease that you can recover from and lead a happy, healthy and productive life. However, if you think that you had to do a little bit of self seeking and self discovery before jumping into a detox situation, that was a cake walk. Reaching a point of "surrender" and starting the road to recovery requires that you be willing to honestly take a look at yourself and take some action.

Am I Really Done With Benzos?

When you're drowning, you don't say 'I would be incredibly pleased if someone would have the foresight to notice me drowning and come and help me,' you just scream. -John Lennon

Hopefully you asked yourself this question before you put yourself through any sort of detox. What's important to understand here is that for most of us, benzos provided some sort of benefits in the beginning and for potentially a long period of time in our lives. Then, at some point, negative consequences of the drugs started to accumulate and, either it just wasn't fun anymore, it wasn't working anymore, or the consequences were too painful to want to continue using them. Regardless, many of us call this a "bottom" and you should take some time to try to define what your bottom is and how it could (and would) get worse should you continue to use benzos.

Unfortunately, addicts are characterized by extreme arrogance and stubbornness. This is why many of us have multiple "bottoms" - where we stop using and think that we can control our using so decide to give it another try. I can tell you from experience and from observing countless others that things always get worse and that attempts to control an addiction are, in the end, futile. Sometimes deadly. The fact of the matter is this - we can choose our bottom. This can be it - right now.

Story:

I am from a small developing country (Papua New Guinea). I was introduced to lorazepam by a kindly local doctor who took pity on the degree of anxiety that I suffered as a result of high school and college experiences of being bullied as well as considerable alcohol and marijuana use during this time. This introduction to lorazepam early in my work career, commenced an addiction for 10 years. When I didn't take it I suffered from a case of shakes and severe neck spasms. Local psychiatrists responded by recommending increased dosages, I eventually found myself buying from the black market and taking 50 x 1mg tablets of black-market lorazepam a day, this cost me a fortune. I lost many career opportunities, and became an alcoholic at age 32. After resigning from a senior managerial position I spent a full year trying to get off this medication as well as alcohol addiction. After a year of going back and forth to the local psychiatric ward, including 2 nights of being admitted to hospital in a semi-conscious state (due to panadol overdose whilst in search of a high), I kicked the lorazepam habit as well as my alcohol addiction. I give a lot of the credit to my faithful wife of 13 years. If anyone out there is experiencing the same, get help, lorazepam addiction can be serious! By the way I have fully recovered now, and am an academic at the local university.

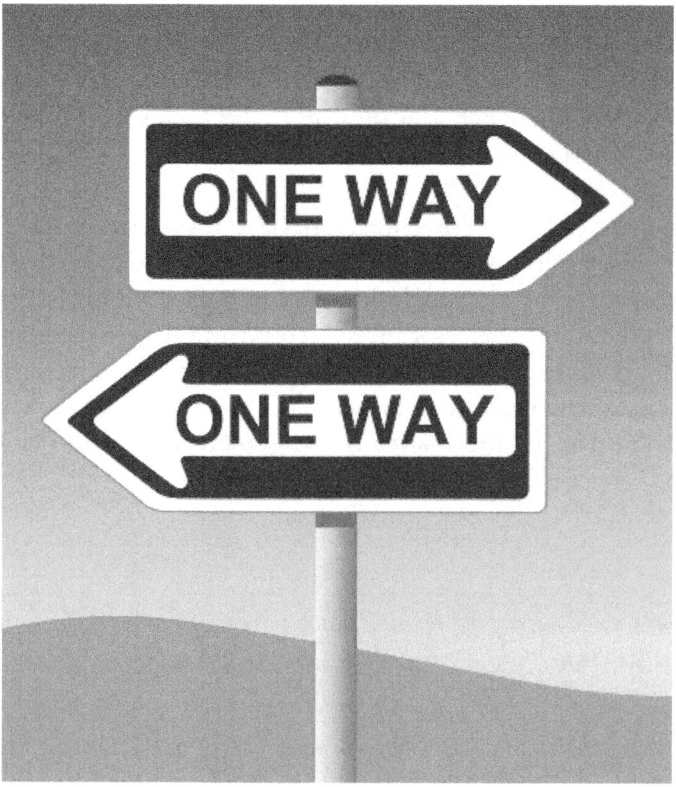

Should I Go to Treatment?

If you want what you've never had, you must do what you've never done.

Most addicts assume that they have to go to treatment to get better. I did and ended up in an endless stream of rehabs. In fact, if you spend any time in front of the television (most do), then we are taught that in order to "get clean", you have to go to rehab. This isn't necessarily the case and the treatment center industry has seen a recent "boom" in the past few decades as getting clean and sober is now all the rage. So, are these fancy places necessary to start your road to recovery? This is hotly debated and the answer is different for each individual. Many people are able to get clean and sober and stay that way with the help of 12 Step programs alone - no rehab. However, in our fast paced society with all of life's demands, treatment centers certainly have carved out their niche in the "getting clean" process and have some very real value.

It may be that you haven't been given a choice. The edict to "go to rehab" could have been handed down by an employer, a family member, or even a judge. If that's the case, the question has been answered for you. Otherwise, if you are still pondering whether or not to go to treatment, there are several different types of treatment centers to choose from and they certainly do have their benefits if you decide to go.

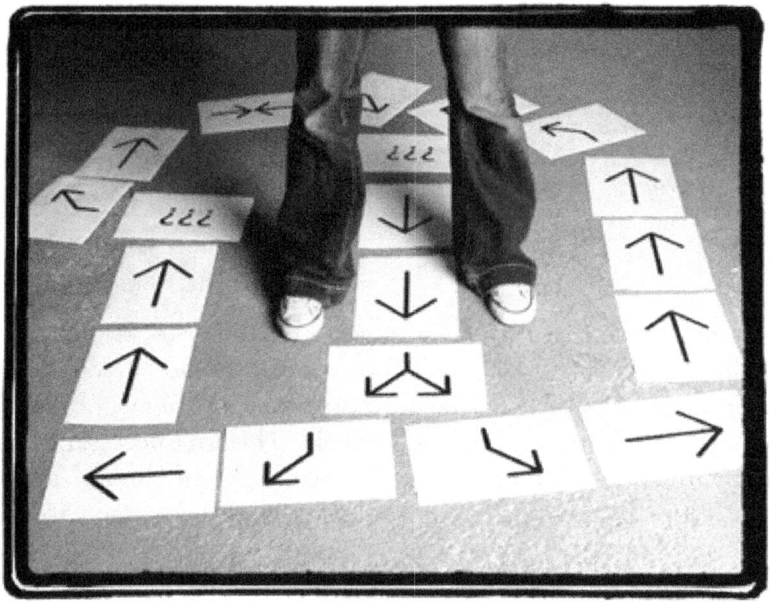

Different Types of Treatment Centers

Choices abound as to what sort of treatment center, if any, is going to be right for you. You will need to decide between Inpatient or Outpatient, Private or Public and, in some cases, Co-Ed or Single Sex treatment centers.

Inpatient vs. Outpatient - Many people are inclined to select "outpatient" right off the bat because we are also inclined to downplay the seriousness of our situation and the means necessary to recover from it. Some people are able to successfully participate in treatment programs on a part-time basis while continuing to live at home, manage their family lives and keep their jobs. These people are exceptions to the rule, however. There are other outpatient treatment programs that simply have you go to treatment during the day and return to your home (and family) at night. Again, depending on your circumstances, this may be a viable option. For many, and for a lot of reasons, it's not for a lot of people.

Inpatient drug and alcohol treatment is more the norm for quite a few reasons. This option dictates that the individual moves into some sort of dorm-like setting and receives 24/7 care and supervision. Some treatment centers allow for private and semi-private rooms, while others you will essentially take what you are given. Inpatient treatment is the ideal choice for someone who needs a place to focus entirely on their addiction and developing their recovery program.

Private vs. Public - Regardless of the previous differences, you will run into rehab centers that are both Private and Publicly funded. Different treatment funding sources include:

- Private: Non-profit, or For Profit
- State or Locally Funded
- Low Cost Treatment Centers
- Free Rehabs (Charity Rehabs)

While the Free, Low Cost and Government Funded treatment centers sound great (they are, I got sober in one), it's important to note that many also have long waiting lists. Another difference, although not true in all cases, may be the size of groups in therapy sessions, with smaller groups in Private facilities and larger groups in publicly funded rehabs. Also, do not expect to get into any sort of private or semi-private room in a public facility. In retrospect, being "pampered" did nothing to get me sober. I did find the many waiting lists very disheartening though when I was finally "ready" for this and just couldn't get in anyplace. So, if you are looking at Private treatment centers and possible ways to finance it, consider these:

- **Health Insurance** - most "good" health insurance policies provide for some form of substance abuse treatment. If you have a really good policy, you may be able to get an inpatient treatment program paid for
- **Family Members** - you may already have family members offering to pay to get you clean. I did. I even had friends of family willing to chip in at one point.
- **Sell stock or take money from your 401k** - If you're unemployed, in jail or dead, there will be no "retirement" to save for, right?
- **Home Equity Loan** - If you are lucky enough to still be holding onto your home, consider this.
- **Sell stuff, even your car** - Chances are you have expensive toys you haven't been using because of you've been putting all of your efforts into drinking and drugging. Sell them. You don't need a car if you're not clean. It's a hazard.
- **Substance Abuse Treatment Loan** - Yes, they have these now.

Co-ed vs. Same Sex Treatment Centers - I've been to both and it didn't make a difference to me either way. However, if you have been the victim of abuse and think that you would feel safer in a same sex facility, by all means, check them out.

The Pros and Cons of Going to Rehab

When I first started hitting the treatment centers, I didn't see any "Pro's" to this nonsense whatsoever. I did not want to be there, did not think that I had a problem like the rest of the folks in that place did and felt very inconvenienced by the whole thing. Quite a few treatment centers and many years of sobriety later, it's much easier to see their benefit. However, I do clearly see what the Con's are in committing to these institutions. Here are a few:

Con's of Going to Treatment

Time - Yes, you are committing a substantial amount of your time to this program. You are committing literally ALL of your time if you elect to go to an inpatient treatment center. This means that family and work responsibilities need to be re-arranged. In many cases, some or all of those have "dissolved" on their own because of our drinking and drugging activities.

Cost - Most people would agree that this is the biggest downside to treatment, particularly private rehabs. Inpatient programs can cost upwards of $1,000 per day and outpatient programs are not cheap either. Publicly funded programs are more affordable but there are oftentimes many hoops to jump through to qualify and get into these programs.

Pro's of Going to Treatment

Structured Environment - One of the biggest benefits of attending treatment, primarily residential (or inpatient), is that you are provided with a safe, structured environment that is free of distractions and temptations. This will give you a window of opportunity to get clean and sober (post-detox) and learn how to live life without drugs and alcohol. This structured environment is designed to essentially be free of the daily stressors of work, home and family so that you can focus only on your recovery.

Establish Network of Positive People - Attending treatment, inpatient or outpatient, gives you the opportunity to form new friendships and bonds with other like-minded, positive people. These are relationships that can be the beginning of your sober support network.

Learning Better Holistic Health - If giving up drugs and alcohol were enough, this would be a much shorter book. However, the real purpose of recovery is to learn how to live a happy and healthy life without drugs and alcohol. Learning to treat yourself well in all respects in something that you can learn in treatment, such as eating right, being physically active and taking care of your mental and spiritual well-being.

Save Money - Wait, what?! Didn't we just say in the "Con's" that "cost" was a downside to going to treatment? Well, yes we did. BUT, let's look at the big picture here. The amount of money that you will save in long run by getting, and staying clean & sober, is astounding compared to continuing with that financial minefield of active addiction. Many people are blown away when they see the financial figures tied to their disease. I'm not just talking about the money spent on drugs and alcohol (count this, though). Add in jobs lost, promotions lost, missed opportunities, legal fees, smashed cars, foreclosed homes, and so on. Looking at it this way, the cost of a stint at that fancy rehab may not look as outrageous as it did earlier.

Save Your Life - For some, it really does boil down to this. It's simply a matter of life or death. Without some real, structured help, the end is imminent. A lot of addicts and alcoholics run to treatment in hopes that they will "save" something or get their lives back. What many find is that they have been given an entirely new life that is infinitely better than anything they could have ever dreamed possible.

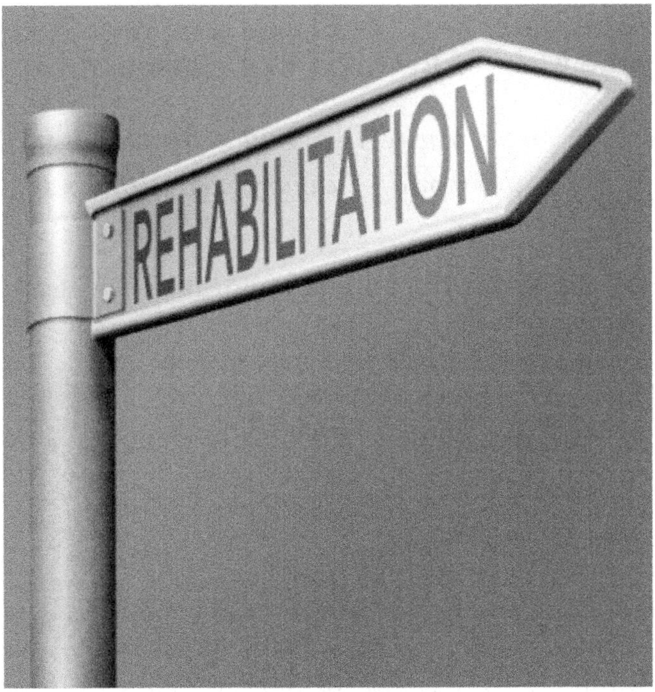
REHABILITATION

Making the Most of Rehab If You Decide to Go

...we do not always like what is good for us in this world. -Eleanor Roosevelt

If you make the decision to go to a treatment facility, good for you! You are giving yourself a gift that will not only come back to you tenfold but to those you know and love as well, even if your relationships aren't as you would want them to be right now. As we reviewed earlier, there are so many different types of treatment facilities so it's not possible to give you a perfect run down of what to expect. However, here are a few words of wisdom so that you can make the most of your stay:

If you have not detoxed from benzos yet, be absolutely sure that the treatment center you choose knows how to do this properly. This means that you will NOT be thrown into a detox facility for seven days and then admitted to the rehab "benzo free". It doesn't work that way. You will need to be in a facility that knows how to do a long, slow, taper from benzos that will most likely continue after your discharge. If you can't find one of those, you may need to put off treatment until you have finished with your taper.

As for the treatment center itself, there will be no locks on the doors. This doesn't work, not even for a second, if you're not willing so you can walk away at any time. Even if you are court ordered to be at a place, they'll just come and pick you up to face your consequences at a later date should you bolt. Check your willingness level at the door, and thereafter frequently, and commit to stay for whatever term is recommended.

If you go - From my experience with the revolving doors of many treatment centers, these are my words of wisdom. First and foremost, check the attitude at the door. This is one thing that I took in with me and held onto through nearly all of my stays, except for the last one. It did me no favors. Thinking that I still knew what was best for me, after the shit storm that I had just made of my life was ludicrous.

Also, demanding that I be given respect and attention when I felt I needed it was just as insane. I had to come to a place where I finally understood that I knew absolutely nothing about how to recover from this disease and that these people were clearly authorities on the subject. So probably, I should just let them do their job and listen to someone else for a change. Once I did this - made this mental shift (some would call it "surrender"), going to treatment was a blessing for me and I made the most of every single opportunity that was put in front of me to learn and to start my recovery. Yes, this included going to AA, which I also resisted for a long time.

The Importance of Joining a Support Group

Separate reeds are easily broken; but bound together they are strong and hard to break apart. -The Midrash

---

Yes, we are talking about a 12 Step Group here, AA or NA preferably. There are alternative "recovery groups" out there but this author knows absolutely nothing about them or their success rates. What I do know is that 12 Step Groups work 100% for people that follow the directions 100%. That's the key. Many people, myself included, have avoided getting sober simply because they feared "joining" AA or NA. I had no concept of what this group was or just how something like this could possibly be of any assistance to me. I didn't understand what AA was and there is always the fear of the unknown.

So, what is AA then? What it is, really, is a multi-faceted program that incorporates meetings, fellowship and working a 12-step program in order to bring about a change in the alcoholic (or addict) and provide continued growth and support. (NA is the same - they just change some words around in the "steps" and the literature is different.) AA was founded in 1935 by Bill Wilson (known as Bill W) and Dr. Robert Smith (known as Dr. Bob), based on the main principle of one alcoholic sharing their experiences with another. Within 4 years, their basic text called "Alcoholics Anonymous" (aka The Big Book) was published and membership blossomed. Today, there are over 2 million members of AA world-wide (over 1/2 of these in the U.S.) and over 115,000 registered AA Groups. In fact, there are now over 200 different fellowships that employ the "12 Steps" for recovery from AA (altered to fit). Hard to argue with those numbers.

Giving up control is difficult and joining a "Support Group" of any sort is giving up another layer of control with respect to this disease. Believe me - I get it. I had to get to a place in my life and with my disease where I finally understood that my way wasn't working in any way, shape or form and I became willing to try something else. Recovery from addiction happens on many levels: physical, mental, emotional and spiritual. The program of AA addresses these different levels of recovery through it's different facets of: attending meetings, getting a sponsor, working the 12 steps, spiritual principles and involvement in the fellowship. In doing these things, old habits are broken, new (healthy) habits are formed, and we are able to take a deeper look at the causes and conditions underlying our long using and/or drinking careers. All of this is done in some manner that taps into the mechanisms that counter the complex neurological and psychological processes through which this disease wreaks its havoc. Better yet, it's done through the power of "the group". Psychologists have long known that one of the best ways to change human behavior is to gather people with similar problems into groups instead of treating them individually. This is one of AA's precepts.

Many people with a prescription drug addiction and find that they simply cannot relate no matter how hard they try. If that's the case, try another 12 Step fellowship. I would venture to suggest that those who continue to focus on how special and unique their situations are will encounter great difficulty in finding that perfect fit, in a 12 Step Group or otherwise. NA or AA is geared toward recovery, period. The type of drug is quite inconsequential. Unless you are too closed minded to find the similarities then a cocaine addict can find recovery in AA if he or she desires (this is my opinion based on what I've seen and experienced over many years). I have found over the years that I can talk about recovery all day and all night without mentioning any substance, because booze and drugs are what recovery *isn't* about. Recovery is about living a good life and doing the next right thing, and that translates the same at any meeting.

John's Story:

I'm now 22 months clean off of Rx Opiates and benzos. I'm active in my local NA group, and I work my program diligently. I lost a very fine teaching career to addiction (after 33 years). I've regained the love of my Family, my self-respect, and a lot of serenity and peace. Rx drug addiction outstrips all other drugs abused in the

U.S., with the exception of alcohol. I find satisfaction in helping others who are going through the hell of addiction. Upscale Rx drug addicts, are (in my experience) the most difficult category of addicts to get into the NA rooms. They are "Addicted" but they aren't "Addicts". The Stigma is so great, they will lose their lives rather than lose their face.

Incidentally, I still have some physical pain (as many Rx opiate addicts do). I can deal with it, far better than I could deal with addiction. I occasionally still have some mild PAWS episodes. However, I recognize them, and that always has helped me deal with them.

Whether it is the initial act of "surrender", the group support setting, the self-awareness that comes from working the Steps, or the close relationships in the fellowship through helping others that are the key components to the addict's recovery (one or all of these), no one knows. What we do know, however, is that despite all we've learned over the past few decades about psychology, neurology, and human behavior, contemporary medicine has yet to devise anything that works markedly better. "In my 20 years of treating addicts, I've never seen anything else that comes close to the 12 steps," says Drew Pinsky, the addiction-medicine specialist who hosts VH1's Celebrity Rehab. While AA or NA may not be a miracle cure for all, people who become deeply involved in the program stay clean & sober and do well over the long haul, and this starts with attending meetings. Check out the Resources Section at the end of the book for links to various 12 Step Groups. It starts by attendance at the first meeting and goes from there. Addiction is not something that can, or should, be battled alone.

"The feeling of having shared in a common peril is one element in the powerful cement which binds us." —Alcoholics Anonymous

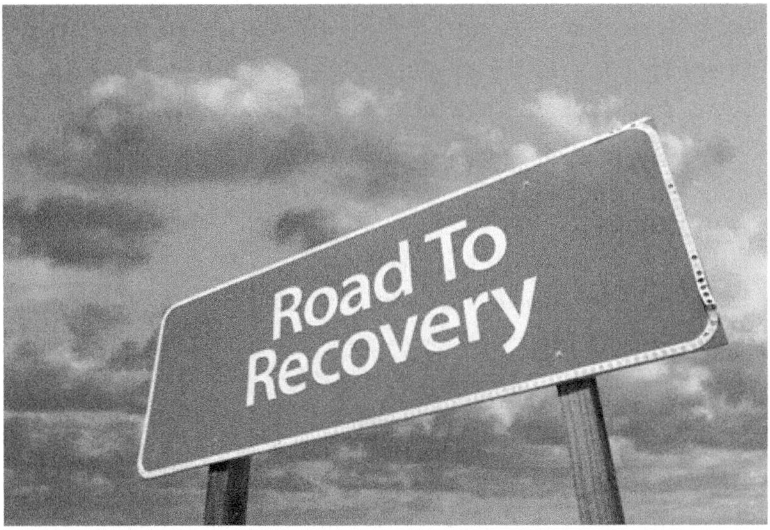
Road To
Recovery

Other Benzo Addiction Considerations

Benzodiazepine addiction, really any addiction, isn't just something that affects the addict. As an addict myself, I remember thinking that I wasn't hurting anyone but myself. This was the furthest thing from the truth. I was having a profound effect on nearly everyone who crossed my path, including family members, employers, friends, and society at large. There are several other influences that we want to take a look at with regards to benzo addiction. These include the effects that we have on our family and loved ones, including some words of advice if you are the loved one being affected. Other considerations are the rise in senior addiction and the role that benzos are playing in this and the role of the family physician in addiction and recovery.

For Family Members

Addicts don't deny that they're using. They deny that it's hurting others. - Bob Poznanovich

Many family members know for fact that there is an addiction issue, while some continue to wish it away or look for any reassurance from the family member in question that things are "ok". Hint: addicts are masters at giving these sorts of reassurances and guarantees, even if they have no idea that they're doing so at the time. So, in order to get rid of the ambiguity, here is a list of questions, from the National Institute on Drug Abuse (NIDA), that you can ask yourself with regards to your loved one:

1. Does the person take the drug in larger amounts or for longer than they meant to?

2. Do they want to cut down or stop using the drug but can't?

3. Do they spend a lot of time getting, using, or recovering from the drug?

4. Do they have cravings and urges to use the drug?

5. Are they unable to manage their responsibilities at work, home, or school, because of drug use?

6. Do they continue to use a drug, even when it causes problems in their relationships?

7. Do they give up important social, recreational or work-related activities because of drug use?

8. Do they use drugs again and again, even when it puts them in danger?

9. Do they continue to use, even when they know they have a physical or psychological problem that could have been caused or made worse by the drug?

10. Do they take more of the drug to get the effect they want?

11. Have they developed withdrawal symptoms, which can be relieved by taking more of the drug? (Some withdrawal symptoms can be obvious, but others can be more subtle—like irritability or nervousness.)

If the answer to just a few of those questions was "yes", there is serious concern about addiction. Now, even in case of iatrogenic, or "accidental" addiction, the answers to quite a few of these questions would still be affirmative. The addict may wish to cut down and find that they cannot, may have difficulty managing some responsibilities, may continue to use the drugs despite symptoms worsening due to their effects, and could be experiencing withdrawal symptoms for a variety of reasons. Drugs that originate in a doctor's office or pharmacy make them no less lethal and when an addict is your spouse, child or parent, determining the course of action can take an added sense of urgency. Fault doesn't come into this and needs to be taken off of the table entirely if you expect to gain the trust of your loved one.

If they want help and wish to get off of benzos, this is great. The best thing to do is to support them on this long road ahead. You may need to help them find a physician who can help with a protracted benzo withdrawal if the original prescribing physician doesn't understand what needs to be done or won't cooperate. There are areas of support that we talk about in the sections of this book on withdrawing from drugs at home. Finally, a source of moral support is one of the most important things that someone in recovery needs.

If your loved one does not recognize that there is a problem or if your concerns are met with anger and denial, there is still hope. Responding with anger usually won't get you very far but it's important for the person addicted to understand that their behavior is no longer healthy and that you don't wish to watch them come to further harm or, even worse, die. If all else fails, an intervention may be helpful in getting them to see the negative effects that drugs have had on their lives and those around them. This is a carefully planned process that involves family and friends of the addicted person, who confront them as a group. This is not done to embarrass them but to get their attention and to get a very important message across. Whether you involve a professional interventionist, counselor or addiction specialist will be up to you. This idea is to give your loved one an opportunity to change directions and make some healthy changes with some clear support.

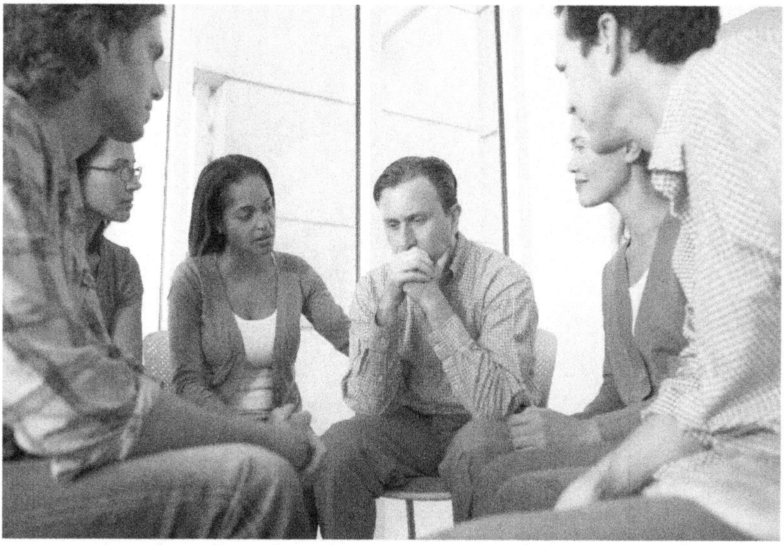

If all else fails, there are now quite a few states that have passed laws allowing for involuntary addiction treatment. This means that, should you be really determined and have a physician's backing, you can petition a judge to force your loved one into treatment. I would only recommend this under the most extreme situations, possibly where benzos were being abused in conjunction with other drugs, making each day of continued use a life threatening situation.

It often seems like those closest to addicts are the ones that suffer the most. I have been the addict that has inflicted the suffering on others and I have been the loved one that has suffered. Neither is a walk in the park and I have much sympathy for both sides. What I have learned through these experiences is that nothing helps to keep an addict sick more than enabling. Once my family members stopped doing this for me, I got better. Therefore, I do my best not to do it for anyone else. This can be a tough, but important, undertaking when you see someone that you love suffering. For more help on these sorts of issues, check out the family support groups in the Resources Section.

Senior Addiction

No one is immune from addiction; it afflicts people of all ages, races, classes, and professions. - Patrick J. Kennedy

Senior addiction is a serious problem in this country and clearly prescription drug addiction is at the heart of that problem. These medications are widely prescribed to the population as a whole but are of particular concern for those patients age 65 and up. A study in JAMA Psychiatry in early 2015 reports that among 65 to 80-year-old Americans, close to 9 percent use one of these sedative hypnotic drugs: Valium, Xanax, Ativan, and Klonopin. Among older women, nearly 11 percent take them. "That's an extraordinarily high rate of use for any class of medications," said Michael Schoenbaum, a senior advisor at the National Institutes of Mental Health (NIMH) and a co-author of the new report.

In 2012, the American Geriatrics Society updated its list of inappropriate medications for older patients and bluntly advised physicians to "avoid benzodiazepines (any type) for treatment of insomnia, agitation, or delirium." The quality of evidence: "High." The strength of the recommendation: "Strong." Not much ambiguity there. Yet when Dr. Schoenbaum and his colleagues dug into a 2008 database that tracked prescriptions at 60 percent of all retail pharmacies in the United States, including mail-order operations, they found benzodiazepine use rising sharply with age. "It just goes up and up," he said. Worse, they found that long-term use also increased with age. Patients of all ages are cautioned to use benzodiazepines for only a few weeks, but in the people aged 65 to 80, nearly a third had taken the drugs for more than 120 days.

It's interesting to note that complications of falls are the leading cause of death among the elderly in industrialized countries. Yet the use of sedatives and sleeping pills increase the risk of falls by about 50%. It has been shown that these drugs are associated with hip fractures, memory problems, increased risk of motor vehicle accidents, and even involuntary urine loss. In 2013, the American Geriatric Society put sedative-hypnotics on its Choosing Wisely list of "Five Things Physicians and Patients Should Question."

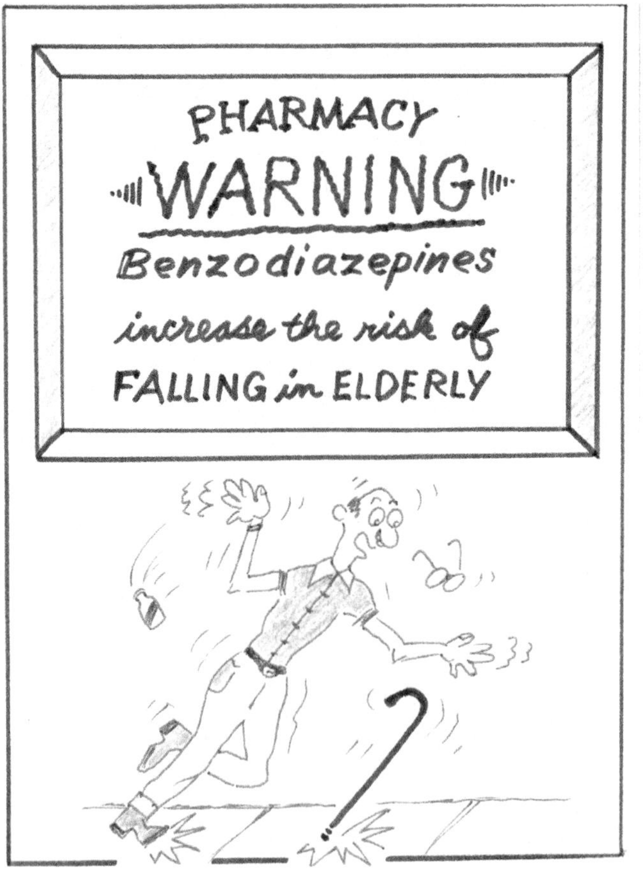

Last summer, the CDC and Johns Hopkins University reported a high number of emergency room visits associated with psychiatric medications in general and Ambien in particular. It looked at visits by age and drug and found the consequences were worse for older people visiting the ER. About a third of those visitors age 65 and older were hospitalized — three times the hospitalization rate for ages 19-44.

Cognitive deterioration associated with normal aging processes and dementia can be worsened by benzodiazepine side effects. Cortical suppression mechanisms may be disturbed in the elderly, and disinhibited behaviors may increase with benzodiazepine use. With less cognitive and social reserve in the elderly patient, the short- and long-term withdrawal symptoms and other benzodiazepine side effects may lead the patient to frequently visit or telephone the physician. The physician may feel "trapped" into arguing against the use of benzodiazepines and prescribing benzodiazepines to elderly patients. In one 1988 study, this impasse was broken by referring elderly patients to inpatient detoxification, which resulted in a dramatic decrease in annual physician visits.

The effects that these drugs can have on elderly patients is scary and pretty frustrating if you or a loved one are over the age of 65 and have been taking them for a prolonged period of time. It is particularly maddening when the patient doesn't feel that there is any reason to make a change. Consider a pilot study that Dr. Gregory Simon, a psychiatrist and senior investigator at the Group Health Cooperative in Seattle, and his colleagues decided to undertake 20 years ago. They planned a program to help people discontinue chronic benzodiazepine use and sent letters announcing it to 50 older patients. "Half the people called and said, 'Don't contact me. I don't want to talk about stopping,'" Dr. Simon recalled. Only five people agreed to discuss the pilot and only two actually showed up.

There IS hope, however, for seniors who have become addicted to benzodiazepines and wish to break free. Family physicians are becoming more educated each day and families themselves are taking control of these situations. There is also some evidence that weaning can be less daunting than patients and physicians believe. A Canadian study has shown that a simple brochure providing a schedule for tapering off the drug over several months can work for some motivated patients, even long-term users. Dr. Simon also recommends the website established by British psychopharmacologist, C. Heather Ashton, that similarly guides users through gradual withdrawal (also linked in our Resources Section).

Mrs. Robinson's Story:

"I am 65 years old and took Lorazepam for 10 years. A few months ago, I fell in the middle of the night on my way to the bathroom and had to go to the hospital. I was lucky and, except for some bruises, I did not hurt myself. I read that Lorazepam puts me at risk for falls. I did not know if I could live without Lorazepam as I always have trouble falling asleep and sometimes wake up in the middle of the night. I spoke to my doctor who told me that my body needs less sleep at my age – 6 hours of sleep per night is enough. That's when I decided to try to taper off Lorazepam. I spoke to my pharmacist who suggested I follow the step-by-step tapering program. I also applied some new sleeping habits I had discussed with my doctor. First I stopped exercising before bed; then I stopped reading in bed, and finally, I got out of bed every morning at the same time whether or not I had a good nights sleep. I succeeded in getting off Lorazepam. I now realize that for the past 10 years I had not been living to my full potential. Stopping Lorazepam has lifted a veil, like I had been semi-sleeping my life. I have more energy and I don't have so many ups and downs anymore. I am more alert: I don't always sleep well at night, but I don't feel as groggy in the morning. It was my decision! I am so proud of what I have accomplished. If I can do it, so can you!'

The Family Physician

Physicians pour drugs of which they know little to cure diseases of which they know less, into humans of whom they know nothing. – Voltaire

When dealing with recovery from benzo addiction, either your own or a loved one's, one of the things that you will need to consider is your future relationship with the source of your drugs. In nearly all cases, the prolonged prescribing of these medications could be considered to be, at the very least, irresponsible. Some may deem it criminal. Unless that physician has been urging you to give up these drugs and warning of their dangers, for years and you've resisted, I'd strongly suggest breaking ties and finding a new doctor. So that there are no questions or temptations later on, I also suggest making that break in writing, letting the physician know that you are leaving because of a prescription drug dependency and do not desire his services in the future. I have done exactly this.

Whether it be a family physician or a psychiatrist, there are those out there who are both conservative and understanding with regards to addiction. To be sure, some psychiatrists are very well versed in the treatment of addiction. Some of the most meaningful contributions to addiction treatment in the 20th century came from psychiatry. Carl Jung's treatment of the intractable alcoholic "Rowland H" led to the foundation of Alcoholics Anonymous. The popular "self-medication" theory of addiction originated in the writings of Edward Khantzian, whose focus on deficient ego strength is informed heavily by psychodynamic theory. And today, the American Board of Psychiatry and Neurology recognizes "Addiction Psychiatry" as a distinct subspecialty, requiring rigorous training, experience in chemical dependency settings, and deep knowledge of substance abuse and its treatment.

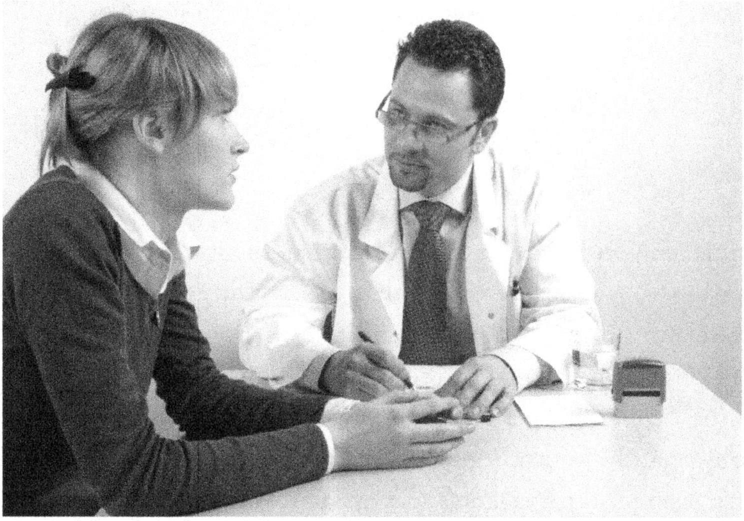

It may take some searches and a few different doctor's visits, but there are good and understanding physicians out there. The most important thing that you will need to do, and it's not always easy, is to speak up immediately about your situation and be honest. There can be no room for a new, overzealous, doctor to whip out his prescription pad and start the madness all over again. You've learned the harm that these medications can render. If you have to educate a few doctors along your journey from here on, so be it.

Life After Benzos

Every tomorrow has two handles. We can take hold of it with the handle of anxiety or the handle of faith. - Henry Ward Beecher

Getting free from benzodiazepines isn't easy and is a long road for many. That being said, most people started taking them in the first place because they had some sort of underlying issue, such as anxiety, insomnia, depression, PTSD, or some other psychosocial disorder. These symptoms often become more pronounced as benzo addiction progresses and withdrawal sets in. Many find that these symptoms will dissipate to varying degrees with time. Others still need some sort of treatment and medication for these disorders and this is where things get tricky if you have just been through one of the most traumatic experiences of your life getting off of drugs.

In this section, we are going to talk about life after benzos. We'll go over the various types of drugs that you definitely need to avoid, alternative medications for these various conditions, and holistic treatments and coping strategies for anxiety.

Medications and Substances to Avoid

Half the modern drugs could well be thrown out the window, except that the birds might eat them. - Martin Henry Fisher

After becoming addicted to one substance, accidentally or not, the chances that you are now susceptible to becoming addicted to others has gone up exponentially. Your brain chemistry has been irrevocably changed and you will need to take this into account with regards to future prescription medications and recreational activities. It would be best to avoid all mood and mind-altering substances from now on. This includes alcohol, marijuana and any other illicit drugs. If you have made the, wise, choice to attend a 12 Step Fellowship for continuing support, you will find your participation much smoother should you decide to do this.

With regards to medication, I am not a physician but it should go without saying that you should never put any sort of benzodiazepine in your system - ever again. Once addicted to a drug, you will ALWAYS be addicted to that drug and taking it again is a recipe for disaster. That being said, if it needs to be taken in an emergency situation or in connection with a surgical procedure, simply be straightforward with the physician about your history. If there is a substitute, they will give you that. If there isn't, the dosage will be controlled for you and you likely won't go home with a six month supply of the stuff.

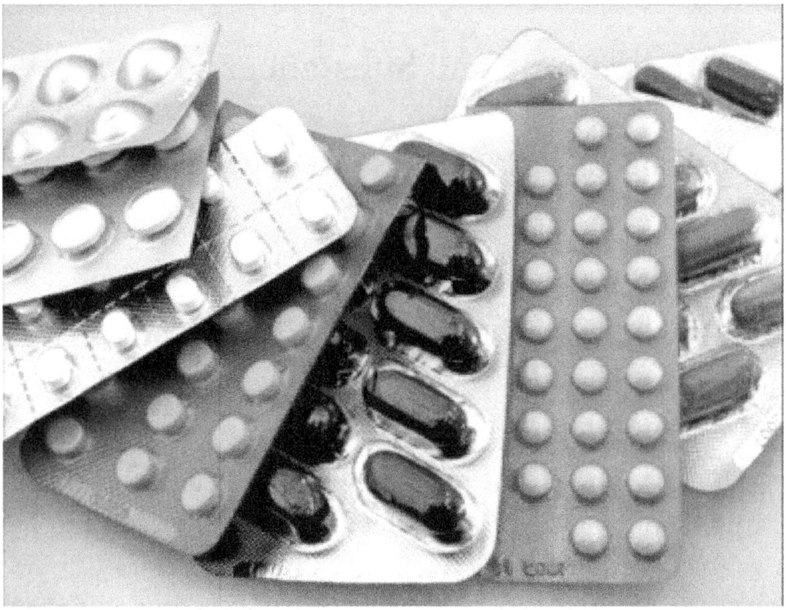

As for medication to be avoided, this becomes difficult because, again, I'm not a physician. Suffice it to say that there are many other prescription medications that are highly addictive and that you may wish to use great caution with. Among these are:

- **Z-Drugs** - These are non-benzodiazepine hypnotics that are prescribed for insomnia. The most popular Z-drugs include zolpidem (Ambien), zopiclone (Zimovane) and zaleplon (Sonata). These drugs are not chemically benzodiazepines but they bind to GABAreceptor complexes which are close to or actually coupled with benzodiazepine receptors. It has been found that the Z drugs produced the same therapeutic and adverse effects as benzodiazepine hypnotics, including tolerance, dependence and abuse.

- **Prescription Opiates** - These medications include: morphine, hydrocodone, fentanyl, methadone, oxycodone, and codeine. Prescription opioids act on the same receptors as heroin and can be highly addictive. People who abuse them sometimes alter the route of administration (e.g., snorting or injecting) to intensify the effect; some even report moving from prescription opioids to heroin. If you have a chronic pain issue that requires ongoing management, be sure to let your physician know about your history with benzos.

- **Stimulants or Analeptics** - While these may not appeal to most of the people that would take a benzodiazepine in the first place, there's no telling what someone is going to take or feel in the future so they're worth mentioning. These include: Adderall and Adderall XR, Dexedrine, Concerta, Focalin and Focalin XR, Meadate CD, Metadate ER, Methylin, Ritalin, Ritalin LA, Vyvanse, and Desoxyn. These may be prescribed for such things as ADD and they are very addictive.

- **Barbiturates** - These are a class of CNS depressants that have similar effects to benzodiazepines. There are still some of these prescribed for such things as headaches, seizures, anxiety, and epilepsy. Some of the more popular barbiturates include: include: Seconal, Amytal, Pentothal, Fiorinal, and Prominal. These are very addictive and abuse of this substance could lead to respiratory arrest, one of the primary causes of death in barbiturate abusers.

- **Others** - A few drugs that tend to get attention by benzo addicts as either aids to withdrawal or substitute treatments yet that really bear further scrutiny are: Remeron (Mirtazapine) and Neurontin (gabapentin). Before you take either one of these, do a good amount of research and know what you're getting into.

Now that you have this growing list of things that you shouldn't take, rest assured that there are still plenty of solutions out there for you, medical and otherwise.

Alternative Medications

The desire to take medicine is perhaps the greatest feature which distinguishes man from animals. - William Osler

---

A vast majority of people that take benzodiazepines started taking them for anxiety and insomnia issues, so that is what we are going to concentrate on here. It is important to note that not all anti-anxiety medications are the same and that there are different classes of drugs used to treat anxiety. Here are some of the drugs that are considered to be non-addictive and often prescribed for the treatment of these disorders:

- **Selective Serotonin Reuptake Inhibitors (SSRIs)** - SSRIs are one of the most commonly used types of medication for anxiety and are often a psychiatrist's first choice when choosing a medication for this purpose. The reason for this is that SSRIs have been proven to be very effective for anxiety, are non-addictive, don't cause memory impairment or interfere with psychotherapy, and have minimal side-effects. When SSRIs do cause side effects, they usually subside within the first week. A notable exception, however, is decreased sexual sensations which occurs in a significant minority of patients. SSRIs work by increasing the amount of signaling between neurons that use a chemical called serotonin to communicate with each other. They are also used to treat depression. The currently available SSRIs are Prozac (fluoxetine), Celexa (citalopram), Lexapro (escitalopram), Zoloft (sertraline), Paxil (paroxetine), and Luvox (fluvoxamine).

- **Serotonin Norepinephrine Reuptake Inhibitors (SNRIs)** - SNRIs do the same thing that SSRIs do but they also increase the amount of signaling between neurons that use a chemical called norepinephrine to communicate with one another. When used to treat anxiety, the benefits and side effects of SNRIs are essentially the same as those for SSRIs. Like the SSRI, the SNRIs take 4 to 6 weeks to reach maximum effect. The three currently available SNRIs are Effexor (venlafaxine), Cymbalta (duloxetine), and Pristiq (desvenlafaxine).

- **Buspirone** - Buspar (buspirone) is a medication that is sometimes used to treat anxiety. Like the SSRIs, buspirone works by influencing the neurons which use serotonin to communicate, but unlike the SSRIs which increase the amount of serotonin available to all serotonin receptors, buspirone affects only one specific subtype of serotonin receptor. An advantage of this selectivity is that buspirone does not cause the sexual side effects sometimes associated with the SSRIs. Like the SSRIs and SNRIs, buspirone may take 4 to 6 weeks to reach maximum efficacy.

- **Hydroxyzine** - Vistaril (hydroxyzine) is another medication that is sometimes used to treat anxiety. Like benzodiazepines, hydroxyzine's effects occur quickly. Unlike benzodiazepines, hydroxyzine is non-habit forming and does not cause tolerance, withdrawal, or memory impairment. The most significant side effect of hydroxyzine is sedation, but this tends to decrease over time. The anti-anxiety effects of hydroxyzine are thought to be due to its blocking of the histamine receptor; however, hydroxyzine appears to be more effective for anxiety than other antihistamines (such as Benadryl) and this may be due to its interaction with a subset of serotonin receptors.

- **Beta blockers**. Brand names: Inderal, Tenormin. These cardiac drugs counteract the effect of adrenaline and alleviate certain anxiety symptoms such as shaking, palpitations, and sweating. These medications should only be used under direct medical supervision, as they reduce blood pressure and slow the heartbeat. Beta blockers are non-habit forming but should not be taken with other pre-existing medical conditions (such as asthma, congestive heart failure, diabetes, vascular diseases, hyperthyroidism, and angina). They are meant to be used for a short term for anxiety and they are not approved by the U.S. Federal Drug Administration (FDA) to treat anxiety, however they are sometimes prescribed for that purpose.

- **Trazodone -** an antidepressant (unrelated to any others) with hypnotic, anxiolytic and analgesic properties. This drug may be useful in treating withdrawal induced insomnia. It is also indicated for fibromyalgia pain.

This is not a complete list of the medications used to treat anxiety and insomnia, and a psychiatrist may opt to use something else depending on the specific circumstances. Furthermore, some of the medications listed above do not have an FDA indication for an anxiety disorder but are included here because they are frequently used off-label for this purpose. Given the large number of medications that are used for anxiety and their sometimes serious side effects, it is important that these medications be used only under the care of a physician.

Holistic Treatment for Anxiety

If you rely solely on medication to manage depression or anxiety, for example, you have done nothing to train the mind, so that when you come off the medication, you are just as vulnerable to a relapse as though you had never taken the medication. - Daniel Goleman

---

The important thing to remember about anxiety disorders is that they were generally brought about by some circumstance or feelings that are not likely to be changed with medication alone. If this entire exercise hasn't taught us anything else, it's that drugs aren't a cure. Medication and supplements can treat some symptoms of anxiety, but will do nothing to change the underlying issues in your life that are making you anxious. If you're anxious because of your relationships, your past, your financial situation, or anything else, drugs won't change that. Therapy, support groups and lifestyle changes will give you more relief than you could imagine.

There are many treatment alternatives to medication, including cognitive-behavioral therapy, which is widely accepted to be more effective for anxiety than drugs. Other effective treatments for anxiety include exposure therapy, talk therapy, meditation, biofeedback, hypnosis, and acupuncture. To overcome anxiety for good, you may also need to make major changes in your life. Lifestyle changes that can make a difference in anxiety levels include regular exercise, adequate sleep, and a healthy diet.

Cognitive Behavioral Therapy

Cognitive behavioral therapy (CBT) is the most widely-used therapy for anxiety disorders. Research has shown it to be effective in the treatment of panic disorder, phobias, social anxiety disorder, and generalized anxiety disorder, among many other conditions.

Cognitive behavioral therapy addresses negative patterns and distortions in the way we look at the world and ourselves. As the name suggests, this involves two main components:

- **Cognitive therapy** examines how negative thoughts, or *cognitions*, contribute to anxiety.

- **Behavior therapy** examines how you behave and react in situations that trigger anxiety.

The basic premise of cognitive behavioral therapy is that our thoughts - not external events - affect the way we feel. In other words, it's not the situation you're in that determines how you feel, but your perception of the situation.

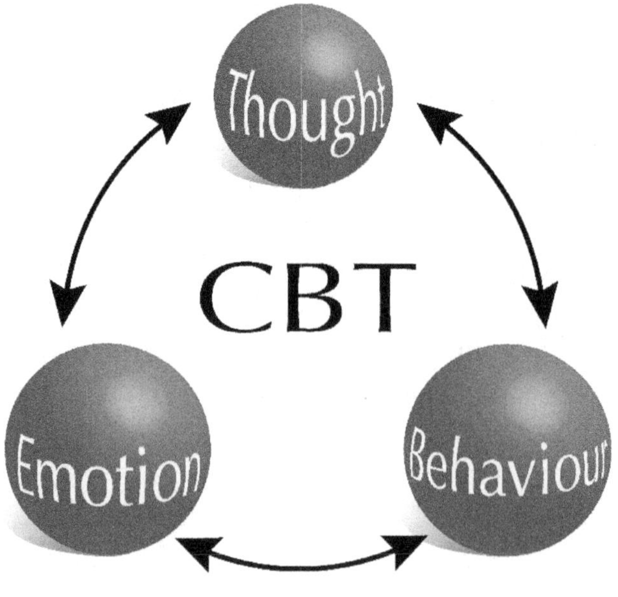

Exposure Therapy

Anxiety isn't a pleasant sensation, so it's only natural to avoid it if you can. One of the ways that people do this is by steering clear of the situations that make them anxious. If you have a fear of heights, you might drive three hours out of your way to avoid crossing a tall bridge. Or if the prospect of public speaking leaves your stomach in knots, you might skip your best friend's wedding in order to avoid giving a toast. Aside from the inconvenience factor, the problem with avoiding your fears is that you never have the chance to overcome them. In fact, avoiding your fears often makes them stronger.

Exposure therapy, as the name suggests, exposes you to the situations or objects you fear. The idea is that through repeated exposures, you'll feel an increasing sense of control over the situation and your anxiety will diminish. The exposure is done in one of two ways: Your therapist may ask you to imagine the scary situation, or you may confront it in real life. Exposure therapy may be used alone, or it may be conducted as part of cognitive behavioral therapy.

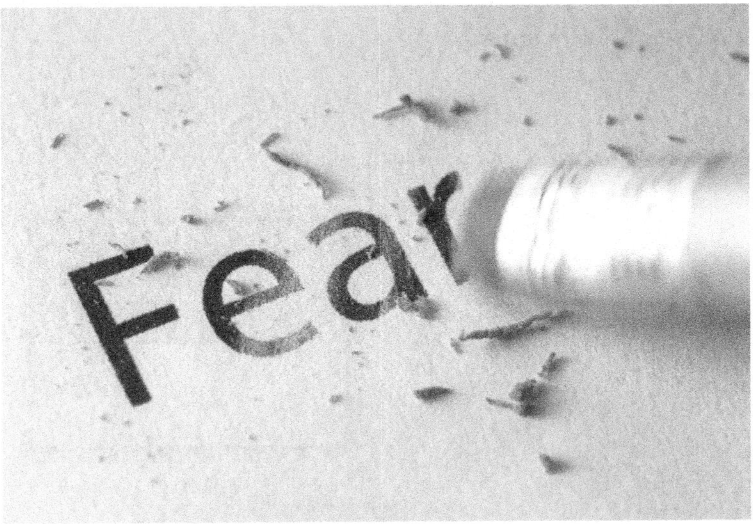

Talk Therapy

Sometimes it's easier to talk to a stranger than to relatives or friends. During talking therapy, a trained therapist listens to you and helps you find your own answers to problems, without judging you. The therapist will give you time to talk, cry, shout or just think. It's an opportunity to look at your problems in a different way with someone who'll respect and encourage your opinions and the decisions you make.

Meditation

When practiced regularly, relaxation techniques such as mindfulness meditation, progressive muscle relaxation, controlled breathing, and visualization can reduce anxiety and increase feelings of relaxation and emotional well-being.

Biofeedback

Using sensors that measure specific physiological functions—such as heart rate, breathing, and muscle tension—biofeedback teaches you to recognize the body's anxiety response and learn how to control them using relaxation techniques.

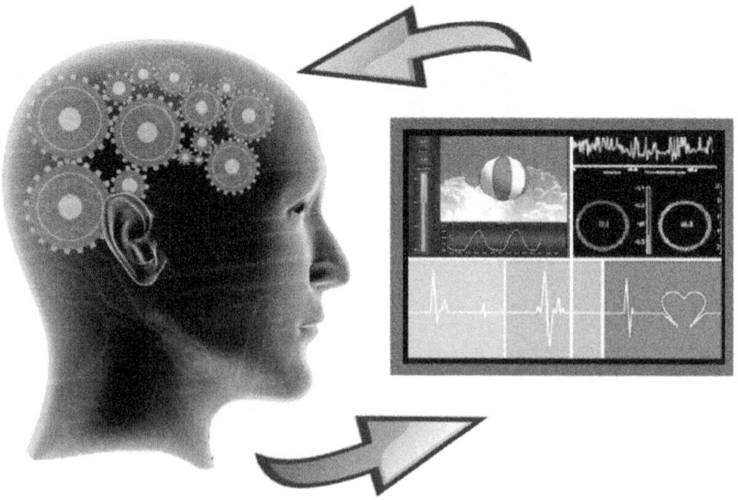

Hypnosis

Hypnosis is sometimes used in combination with cognitive-behavioral therapy for anxiety. While you're in a state of deep relaxation, the hypnotherapist uses different therapeutic techniques to help you face your fears and look at them in new ways.

Acupuncture

In a comprehensive literature review appearing in a recent edition of CNS Neuroscience and Therapeutics, it was proved that acupuncture is comparable to cognitive-behavioral therapy (CBT), which psychologists commonly use to treat anxiety (Errington-Evans, 2011). Unlike with counseling, people treated with acupuncture often see results after one session, and the results improve with continued treatment.

Traditional Chinese medicine relates anxiety to an imbalance of the heart and kidney. Fire represents the heart and joy according to the five elements. The diagnosis is that too much heat in the heart will imbalance the interaction with the kidney (represented as water and fear). This will result in the water organ failing to contain the fire organ rising up to the mind, leading to anxiety. Acupuncture on points around the heart, kidney, spleen and ear are used to treat anxiety.

Exercise

Exercise may be the furthest thing from your mind when going through a long, drawn-out, detox from benzos but it could be one of the things that could benefit you the most. Exercise is not only a natural stress buster and anxiety reliever, but it literally helps to re-train your brain to release dopamine and other "feel good" chemicals on its own. Research shows that as little as 30 minutes of exercise three to five times a week can provide significant anxiety relief. We talked about meditation just a few pages back and you can certainly combine your meditation practices with your exercise routine, particularly if you were to get involved in something as beneficial as yoga.

Sleep

Sleep may be a difficult endeavor in the early months of benzo recovery. Just know that it will continue to get better. There were suggestions in the previous chapter in reference to some safer meds for anxiety and insomnia. Most opt to take nothing new and that's a pretty safe route to travel for many. There are generally recognized tips on getting a good night's sleep that may be of benefit. These include: Setting a regular bedtime and wake up time to establish a regular sleep schedule, get the proper amount of natural light exposure each day, don't eat big meals or drink caffeine before bedtime, get plenty of exercise, and learn to meditate.

Nutrition

It's hard to believe that what we eat could have an effect on our anxiety level but this has been shown to be the case. It makes sense actually. What you eat affects how you feel, and if how you feel is anxious, it stands to reason that changing your diet to one that is made for those living with anxiety can be a valuable part of treating your anxiety symptoms.

It starts by avoiding foods that may contribute to your anxiety symptoms. If you really want to create a diet for anxiety, remove or moderate all of the following: Fried foods, alcohol, coffee (and other caffeinated drinks), excess dairy products, and refined sugars. There are several foods that may reduce your anxiety symptoms. Remember, healthy eating leads to healthy hormonal functioning, which leads to an improved sense of well-being. So the better you eat, the better your anxiety will be. Good foods include: Fresh fruit, vegetables, water, Tryptophan rich foods, Magnesium rich foods, Omega-3 Fatty Acids.

Unless you improve your diet, you're making it harder to reduce anxiety. Anxiety isn't directly linked to diet, but your diet is a contributing factor to both the experience and the severity. Since eating a healthier diet is also important for your health and your self-esteem, changing your diet when you suffer from anxiety makes a great deal of sense. Then you can pair your anxiety diet up with an effective treatment technique.

Practically everybody knows what it's like to feel anxious, worried, nervous, afraid, uptight, or panicky. Often, anxiety is just a nuisance, but sometimes it can cripple you and prevent you from doing what you really want with your life. But I have some great news for you: You can change the way you feel. - David D. Burns

Benzo Recovery Success Stories

I have come to accept the feeling of not knowing where I am going. And I have trained myself to love it. Because it is only when we are suspended in mid-air with no landing in sight, that we force our wings to unravel and alas begin our flight. And as we fly, we still may not know where we are going to. But the miracle is in the unfolding of the wings. You may not know where you're going, but you know that so long as you spread your wings, the winds will carry you. - C. JoyBell C.

I understand that a lot of the material covered in this book may be construed as negative or "depressing" by some. It was meant to be an honest and forthright look at benzodiazepine addiction and to give a clear path to recovery through withdrawal options and then life after detox. Despite the tone of much of the material, there is no doubt that many have beaten this addiction and have gone on to live happy and useful lives. I am one of those people. There are many others and this last section is a collection of stories of other people's successes in breaking free from benzo addiction.

Disclaimer: The success stories contained here have been taken from a variety of sources. Their presence here is in no way a claim of ownership. As such, the names of authors of these stories have been excluded. All stories have been extracted from the original source as verbatim as possible in order to retain the author's intent and meaning to the greatest extent possible. Misspellings, typos, punctuation, and grammar have not been corrected.

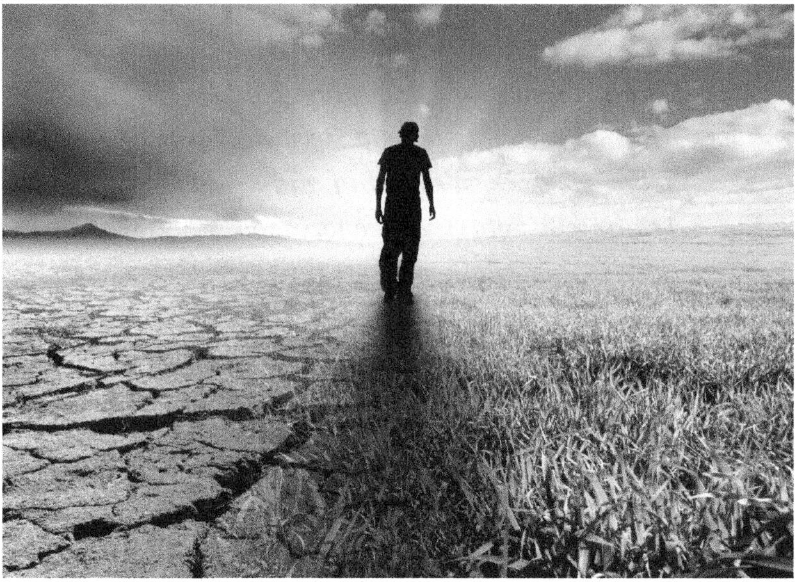

Success Story 1:

At age 30 I was prescribed Temazepam for insomnia. At age 50 I was prescribed 0.25 mg Xanax for (minor) job stress. In 2003 my mother was brutally beaten in a home invasion. She died after a hellish five weeks in ICU at Stanford. Three subsequent murder trials and a divorce found me on a much higher dose of Xanax and several antidepressants. Xanax was the only thing that could stop the crying. A few years later my GP, a truly wonderful and compassionate man, said Xanax wasn't his favorite drug and suggested I switch to something else. I told him it was working great (I thought it was) and he didn't push it. We were both somewhat at fault at this point. I stopped taking Temazepam without tapering. At 2 mg a day, I could hardly stay awake at the end of each day as it was. Xanax probably covered any withdrawal. I taught kindergarten successfully during these years and retired in 2000. With no job stress and my grief manageable, I couldn't figure out why I still needed to take Xanax…I knew I needed the relief it gave me but I had NO idea it was due to physical dependence. I started 'testing', playing around with the Xanax to see if it was actually the cause of the problems or if I was just a hopeless emotional wreck that had to take meds to stay calm. Then I "googled" benzodiazepines. OMG. I started tapering in August 2011 on my own. My cuts were here and there because I didn't know how to properly taper. I realized I had to hold during stressful times like holidays. By Feb 2012 I was down to 0.25mg with relative ease compared to what was coming next. A marriage/drug counselor friend told me to jump. So I did. Three days later I was in full blown withdrawal and felt I had to either reinstate (every fiber of my being resisted taking any more Xanax ever) or die from withdrawal...I KNEW I was in big trouble. I reinstated to 0.25mg and felt immediate relief from the worst of the symptoms.

Finished my taper April 8th,2012 and began immediately to improve. The perpetual headache went away the first day off. The rest were slower to go. The cog fog and memory issues took a while to improve. I also had insomnia, light and sound sensitivity and a host of other minor complaints like burning skin, tremor, dislike for showering, changing clothes, seeing people, fear of driving and stores...But they're gone now. A year later I am doing well. I am increasingly active, I can think and remember, I want to go places, do things and be with other people. Life is good and getting better all the time.

I've been asked why I've recovered so quickly. I think a huge part is that I didn't have to work, didn't have to take care of children. I only took care of myself (I could barely do that). I was able to keep stress down and let healing happen. I have really put myself first in this.

*** Every single symptom (except insomnia and general agitation) was brought on when I went too fast. GO SLOW...if you're not already suffering, DON'T BRING IT ON by rushing your taper. You are not going to kick the benzo's butt, it will kick yours if you rush your taper!*

Success Story 2:

I just wanted to let everyone know, you can heal from this nightmare! At 18 months I realized my complete healing! My w/d sxs were so severe that I could not even fathom there would be an end to it. I am here to say that I am able to ingest absolutely anything I choose too. I have no supplement, RX, food or otherwise reactions or sensitivities to anything anymore, and at one point I could take almost nothing after this started. They are all gone! I had my Gallbladder taken out 6 months ago, outside of telling them no Benzo's or anything related, I came through the surgery with flying colors! No side effects or adverse reactions. My life is back to normal and I lead a normal life. Oh and I can sleeeeeep! I of course will still always take it slow with meds, just because of the knowledge I have learned from this experience. But I no longer live in fear every time I need to take medication or supplements of any sort. The fear no longer hangs in the back of my head. So hang in there, you will recover!

Success Story 3:

I went cold turkey off 1mg of Ativan after only taking them for two months, and descended into an unimaginable hell that took all that God gave me to fight through, but I did, and so will you because the same God that made me, made you also. I'm okay now, I feel like me, and that was one of my biggest fears, would I ever feel like me again. Stay the course, give your brain the time it needs to heal.

Success Story 4:

It's been just over a year since I finished a 4 ½ month taper of Klonopin. It was absolutely the most difficult thing that I have ever encountered in my life and there were a few times when I thought I might be better off dead. I am here to say that I feel, at this point, that I am 100% or so close to 100% that it's insignificant. I tapered directly from Klonopin. It was a slow process. When I got down to 0.5 mg (1 tablet), I cut 1/16th of a tablet each time. Once I finished my taper, things began to improve a lot and it just got better and better. It took a full year to be 100% but even after a month off I saw significant improvement. A few months ago I was still having restless legs, muscle aches, but I just realized a few days ago that they were gone. I hadn't noticed that they were gone because they went away so very slowly. My energy has really returned to normal. It took about nine months for my energy to return to normal. My sensitivities also seem to be improving. I have a daily cola now and tolerate it well. I still can't tolerate sugar, but then I always was somewhat sensitive to sugar. It might be a little worse now but I don't know that I can blame the benzos since I am also entering menopause.

I really wondered if I would ever totally heal, but I did. Once my symptoms were completely gone, I found that I was no longer reading the Benzo Group posts. I do correspond with several members of the group who are still tapering but I no longer feel the strong connection that I once did with the Benzo Group. I think this is a real problem in that the Group needs to hear that healing does happen. I am here to say that I am proof. It takes a load of patience, but it does happen.

Success Story 5:

Please listen to me and believe me. I was on benzos from age 17 to 35. By the time I realized I had to get off of them, I was on 90 mg of temazepam daily and from there switched to 40 mg Valium for a year-long taper. I went into withdrawal about a week after my taper was done. I thought withdrawal would kill me, and it lasted for over two years. Over the first year and a half, it progressively got worse. I couldn't think at all. I was in bed for over a year, only getting up to use the bathroom. My body was made of rubber and full of constant humming and burning. I had the chills for close to two years. Any little noise made me feel like I had just been in an auto wreck. I can go on forever, but all I want to say is I finally got over it and I don't ever remember feeling so good. Ever. Hang in and realize it is going to take a while, but it will go away.

Afterward

Expose yourself to your deepest fear; after that, fear has no power, and the fear of freedom shrinks and vanishes. You are free. —Jim Morrison

---

Breaking free from benzo addiction is a difficult thing, both for the addict and those close to them. I was a person who had to have something to change the way they felt for many years, not understanding that the pills and the alcohol weren't the solution I believed them to be. The drugs that I was taking, in the beginning for legitimate symptoms, were no longer working for me and, in fact, were manifesting many of those original symptoms in a rebound effect. In the end, I was in a dark hole of physical, emotional and some other pretty scary consequences and looking for a way out.

Most addicts don't believe that there is a solution for them, until they are backed up against a wall and have no choice but to try something different. My hope for you, or your loved one, is that this day has come with respect to benzos or any other drug that is ruling your existence. From my own experience, and that of many others that I have met over the years, I can promise you that there IS a solution and it is infinitely better than a life of being tied to any substance. There may be some pain and trials at the beginning, but it will be so worth it in the end. My best to you and your family as you begin your journey back into the light. - Taite A.

Resources

Benzo Resources

The Ashton Manual (http://benzo.org.uk/)
benzo.org.uk is dedicated to sufferers of iatrogenic benzodiazepine tranquilliser addiction. Launched on July 6, 2000, this web site has always been a work in progress consisting of articles, information, expert medical documents, news stories and personal accounts.

BenzoBuddies.org (http://www.benzobuddies.org/)
With nearly 15,000 members, mostly in the U.S., the site was launched in 2004 by a British man, Colin Moran, after his withdrawal from Klonopin. Online members trade their stories and share successes, pointing to "benzo-wise" doctors and discussing the pitfalls of trying to withdraw.

Benzodiazepine Support
(http://www.benzosupport.org/index.htm)
The Benzo Withdrawal support site was developed in association with the online support group called the Yahoo Benzo Group to give easy access to the information which this group had gathered to help people in their journey off benzodiazepines.

Benzo Wise Doctors and Therapists
(http://www.benzodocs.com/)
This is a compiled list (possibly dated) of doctors and therapists world-wide who have been helpful to patients who are trying to stop taking benzos.

Mad in America (http://www.madinamerica.com/)
A site designed to serve as a resource and a community for those interested in rethinking psychiatric care in the United States and abroad.

Treatment Centers

There are no "public" websites that offer treatment center, detox and sober living directories. Unfortunately, any site you find will be filled with "sponsored results". This means rehabs that have paid for ad space. That's not always a bad thing, just not an unbiased thing. The best site I've found is **Sober.com**. You'll get the sponsored results in your search but you will also get all of the public listings as well, including the government-funded (some free) facilities.

Another Treatment Center Resource (http://www.drugrehabcenters.org/ByState/Drug_Rehab_Centers_With_Sliding_Scale_Fees.htm) - This one also lists the treatment centers that either have a sliding fee scale, accept public funds or are free.

Support Groups

Narcotics Anonymous (http://www.na.org/)
Alcoholics Anonymous (http://aa.org/)
Cocaine Anonymous (http://ca.org/)
Nar-Anon Family Groups (http://www.nar-anon.org/naranon/)
Al-Anon Websites (http://www.al-anon.alateen.org/)
Families Anonymous (http://www.familiesanonymous.org/)
Children of Addicts (http://mdjunction.com/children-of-addicts)
Co-Dependence Anonymous (CoDA) (http://www.coda.org/)

Mental Health

National Institute of Mental Health (http://www.nimh.nih.gov/)
Results of biomedical research on mind and behavior.

National Alliance for the Mentally Ill (http://www.nami.org/)
Support for consumers with mental illness

Substance Abuse & Mental Health Services Administration
(http://www.samhsa.gov/)
United States Department of Health & Human Services

Government Resources

Single-State Agency (SSA) Directory:
(http://www.recoverymonth.gov/Recovery-Month-Kit/Resources/Single-State-Agency-SSA-Directory.aspx)
Prevention and Treatment of Substance Use and Mental Disorders – A list of State offices that can provide local information and guidance about substance use and mental disorders, treatment, and recovery in your community.

AMVETS (http://www.amvets.org/)
This organization provides support for veterans and the active military in procuring their earned entitlements. It also offers community services that enhance the quality of life for this Nation's citizens.

Professionals

Intervention Project for Nurses (http://www.ipnfl.org/)
Help for professionals with chemical dependencies.

International Lawyers in Alcoholics Anonymous (ILAA)
(http://www.ilaa.org/)
This organization serves as a clearinghouse for support groups for lawyers who are recovering from alcohol or other chemical dependencies.

International Pharmacists Anonymous (IPA)
(http://home.comcast.net/~mitchfields/ipa/ipapage.htm)
This is a 12-step fellowship of pharmacists and pharmacy students recovering from any addiction.

Other

This Center for Substance Abuse Prevention widget (http://www.samhsa.gov/about/csap.aspx) includes a variety of updates on activities relating to underage drinking which is updated regularly with local, state, and national articles published by online sources.

NCADD: (http://ncadd.org/)
The National Council on Alcoholism and Drug Dependence, Inc. (NCADD) and its Affiliate Network is a voluntary health organization dedicated to fighting the Nation's #1 health problem – alcoholism,

drug addiction and the devastating consequences of alcohol and other drugs on individuals, families and communities.

American Council for Drug Education (http://www.acde.org/)
Educational programs and services for teens, parents, and educators

Faces & Voices of Recovery:
(http://www.facesandvoicesofrecovery.org/)
Faces & Voices of Recovery is dedicated to organizing and mobilizing the over 23 million Americans in recovery from addiction to alcohol and other drugs, our families, friends and allies into recovery community organizations and networks, to promote the right and resources to recover through advocacy, education and demonstrating the power and proof of long-term recovery.

About the Author

Taite Adams grew up everywhere. The only child of an Air Force navigator and school teacher, moving around became second nature by grade school. By age 20, she was an alcoholic, drug addict and self-proclaimed egomaniac. Pain is a great motivator, as is jail, and she eventually got sober has found peace and joy in this life beyond measure.

At the age of 42, Taite published her first book titled "Kickstart Your Recovery". Now permanently Free on Amazon, the book answers many of the questions that she herself had but was afraid to ask before giving up the fight with addiction and entering recovery over a decade prior. Since, she has published four other recovery books, including her bestselling book on Opiate Addiction, and has moved into the broader spirituality and self-help genres.

Leading a spiritual life is all about choices. The practice of spiritual principles and the willingness to remain teachable are the key ingredients for growth. As a spiritual seeker and reader of the self-help genre herself, Taite appreciates and respects each and every person who takes the time to read her works and respond with reviews and comments. For more information on books, upcoming releases, and to connect with the author, go to http://www.taiteadams.com.

Check out our active Facebook Page: Taite Adams.

As you begin your Road to Recovery, please check out Taite's first book, Kickstart Your Recovery, available in both Kindle (where's it is Permanently FREE) and Paperback.

Should you require additional assistance with your home detox, be sure to pick up Taite's popular book, Safely Detox From Alcohol and Drugs at Home, also on Amazon.com.

Opiate Addiction has reached epidemic proportions in this country and is something that Taite is intimately familiar with. Read her bestselling book on this topic, chronicling this insidious killer and laying the pathway for freedom from its grip.

If you or a loved one are in recovery from alcoholism or addiction and want to learn more about emotional sobriety, check out Taite's book titled Restart Your Recovery, also on Amazon.com.

It's hard to miss mention in the media of the drug Molly and the controversy surrounding it's use and it's ingredients. There is plenty of confusion there as well. Check out Taite's latest book, called Who is Molly? for the latest info on this drug and it's dangers.

Have you ever wanted to learn more about Ego? Taite's latest book, titled E-Go: Ego Distancing Through Mindfulness, Emotional Intelligence & The Language of Love, takes an in depth look at ego. Consider how you define yourself and how to live a happier life, apart from ego in your career, relationships, and health.

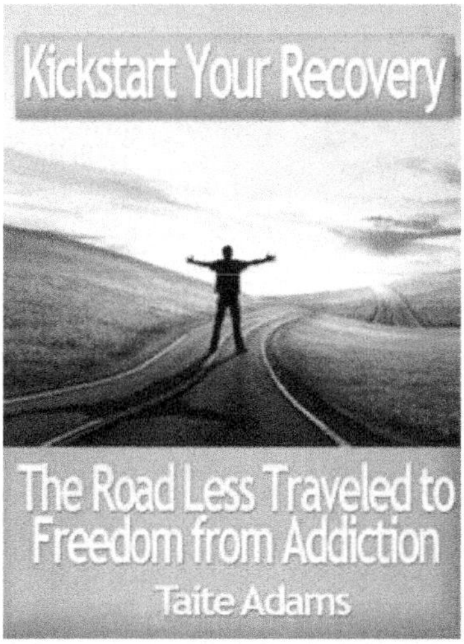
Kickstart Your Recovery
The Road Less Traveled to Freedom from Addiction
Taite Adams

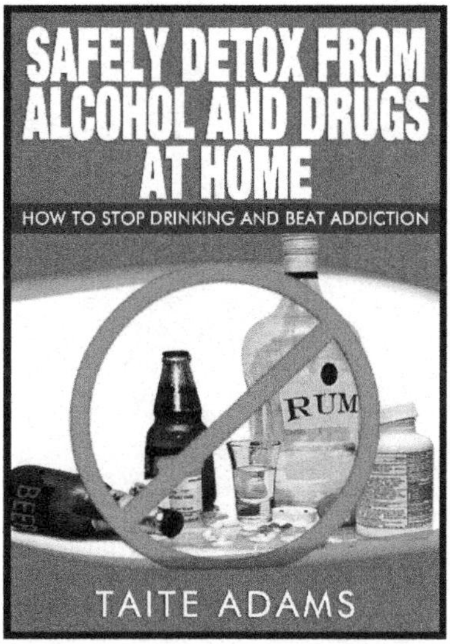
SAFELY DETOX FROM ALCOHOL AND DRUGS AT HOME
HOW TO STOP DRINKING AND BEAT ADDICTION
RUM
TAITE ADAMS

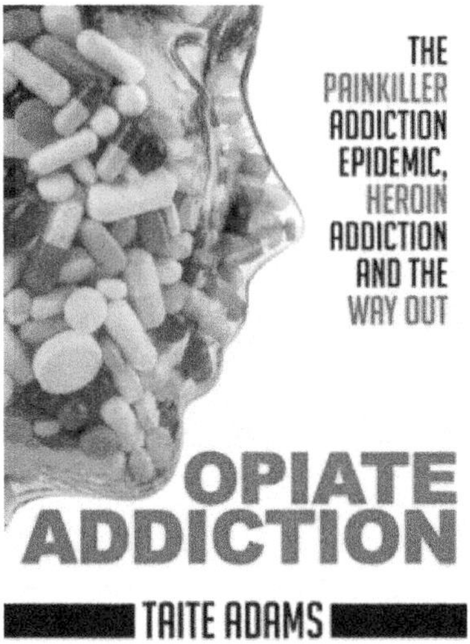
THE
PAINKILLER
ADDICTION
EPIDEMIC,
HEROIN
ADDICTION
AND THE
WAY OUT
OPIATE
ADDICTION
TAITE ADAMS

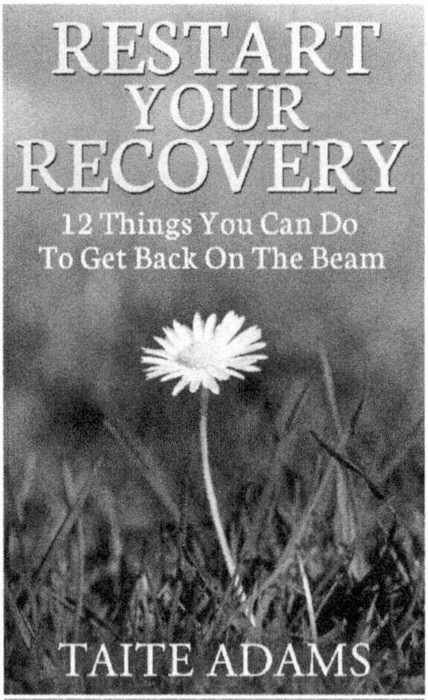
RESTART
YOUR
RECOVERY
12 Things You Can Do
To Get Back On The Beam
TAITE ADAMS

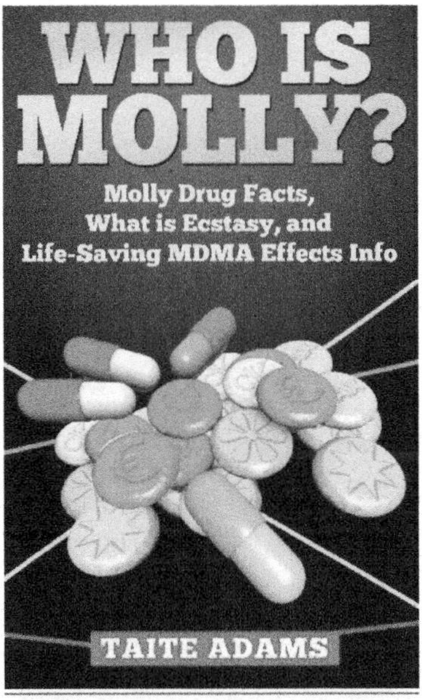
WHO IS
MOLLY?
Molly Drug Facts,
What is Ecstasy, and
Life-Saving MDMA Effects Info
TAITE ADAMS

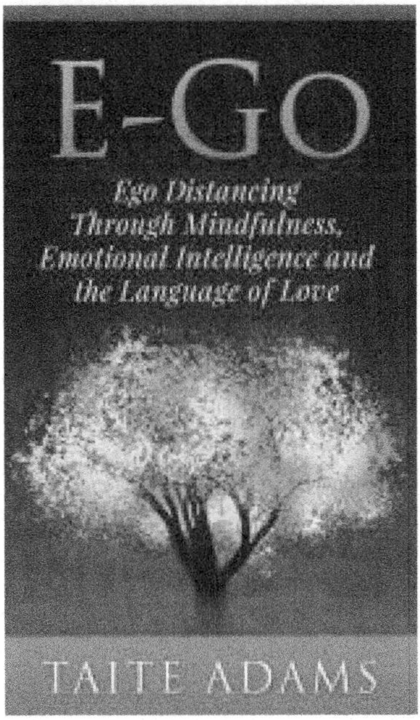
E-GO
Ego Distancing
Through Mindfulness,
Emotional Intelligence and
the Language of Love
TAITE ADAMS

Beyond Benzos

26143855R00116

Made in the USA
Middletown, DE
18 December 2018